A variety of exercise programme
and physical fit.

THE
CHINESE
ART OF
EXERCISE
FOR A
HEALTHY
AND
LONG LIFE

THE CHINESE ART OF EXERCISE FOR A HEALTHY AND LONG LIFE

DAHONG ZHUO M.D.

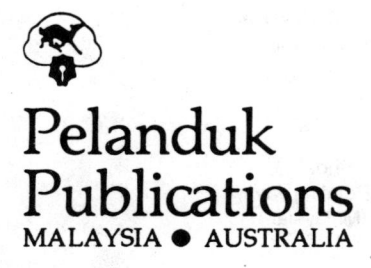

Pelanduk Publications
MALAYSIA ● AUSTRALIA

Published in 1989 by
Pelanduk Publications (M) Sdn Bhd.
24 Jalan 20/16A, 46300 Petaling Jaya,
Selangor Darul Ehsan, Malaysia.

All rights reserved.
Copyright © 1989 by Dahong Zhuo M.D.
Illustrations copyright © by Hartley & Marks Ltd..
Cover art copyright © 1989 by Pelanduk Publications.
This book may not be reproduced in whole or in part, by mimeograph or any other means, without permission from the Publisher.

Reprinted 1991

Published by arrangements with
Hartley & Marks Ltd, 3663 West Broadway,
Vancouver, B.C., Canada.

First published by Harley & Marks Ltd, as
The Chinese Exercise Book.

Perpustakaan Negara Malaysia
Cataloguing-in-Publication Data

Zhua, Dahong
The Chinese art of exercise for a healthy
and long life/Dahong Zhua.
ISBN 967-978-285-9
1. Exercise therapy – China. 2. Physical
fitness. 3. Therapeutics, Physiological.
I. Title.
615.820951

Printed by
Eagle Trading Sdn Bhd.
81 Jalan SS25/32, 47301 Petaling Jaya,
Selangor Darul Ehsan, Malaysia.

CONTENTS

PREFACE 7
HOW TO USE THIS BOOK 11

PART I
TRADITIONAL CHINESE EXERCISES

Introduction 17
1 *Tai Chi Chuan* 19
2 *Yi Jin Jing* — Muscle Strengthening Exercises 35
3 *Ba Duan Jin* — Eight Fine Exercises 49
4 *Shier Duan Jin* — Twelve Fine Exercises 59
5 *Chi Kung* — Invigorating Exercises 65
6 Other Traditional Chinese Exercises 77

PART II
CHINESE FITNESS EXERCISES

7 Fitness Exercises for Children 83
8 Fitness Exercises for the Sedentary 89
9 Fitness Exercises for the Elderly 97
10 Fitness Exercises for Pregnant Women 105
11 Fitness Exercises for Athletes 111

CONTENTS

PART III
CHINESE THERAPEUTIC EXERCISES

12	Exercises for Hypertension	121
13	Exercises for Arteriosclerosis	131
14	Exercises for Coronary Heart Disease	135
15	Exercises for Gastrointestinal Problems	159
16	Exercises for Anxiety and Depression	167
17	Exercises for Insomnia	171
18	Exercises Following Brain Concussion	173
19	Exercises for Paralysis	175
20	Exercises for Sciatica and Lumbar Disk Problems	187
	INDEX	193

PREFACE

In this modern age, the critical need for exercise therapy is especially felt when "life on wheels" and work with machines give us convenience and comfort at the cost of our health. The so-called diseases of civilization, or hypokinetic diseases, such as coronary heart disease and obesity have become epidemic. In part, at least, their origin may be traced to lack of activity, and appropriate, regular exercise will do much to prevent them. In addition, with numerous new drugs appearing on the market each year, many patients and physicians tend to rely on medication, while fundamental recovery through therapeutic exercise is neglected. Clearly, the health and happiness of chronic patients and their families will be enhanced by a knowledge of exercise therapy. A popular scientific book on this topic is a necessity today.

However, during my recent visit to North America, I was happy to find that, with the development of the holistic approach to health care in recent years, there has been a growing interest in Oriental preventive and therapeutic methods. Among those being brought to the attention of North Americans are programs of Chinese exercise therapy such as *Tai Chi Chuan* and *Chi Kung*, to mention only two of the most valuable.

Indeed, Chinese exercise methods are going to the West, and well deserve to do so. Chinese exercise carries a tradition of over 2,500 years. Numerous accounts found in medical classics and historical writings have shown its usefulness in maintaining health and promoting longevity. What is more important is that Chinese exercise therapy is now coming of age. The exercise programs which are widely used in China today represent a refinement of the ancient tradition. Over the past three decades Chinese clinical and experimental research has proved the effectiveness of Chinese therapeutic exercise and has revealed its underlying physiological mechanisms. Today the application of this kind of exercise therapy is guided by physiological and medical principles, thereby increasing the benefits to the patient. However, despite recent innovations, Chinese exercise programs still retain many unique traditional characteristics. It is this tradition which makes Chinese exercise therapy distinctive and gives it so much of its value.

Generally speaking, the Chinese systems of therapeutic exercise are characterized by slow and gentle movements with representative or symbolic implications, mental concentration during performance of the exercise, and the adjunctive application of self-administered massage. Physiologically and psychologically oriented, they have been found to be beneficial in chronic diseases, as well as where there are psychosomatic factors, and for preventive health in general. Most of the Chinese traditional exercise programs may be regarded as body/mind or body/image techniques, since both the body and the mind are trained during the practice. As a consequence, not only are the muscles, heart, and lungs strengthened, but the psychological and emotional states are also enhanced, promoting harmony and balance between body and mind. In this connection, I join many a physician of the West in suggesting that in today's world of hurried living and stress, these unique and ancient exercises may be a source of relaxation and peace of mind. They offer patients a means of relieving tension and shortening the recovery phase of long-term illness, particularly in diseases with a psychosomatic component, such as hypertension and peptic ulcer, as well as the psychoneuroses.

In addition, Chinese exercise therapy is effective in improving physical fitness and general well-being. It is well known that the middle-aged and elderly can benefit a great deal from the gentle movements of Chinese exercise. However, younger people — children as well as teenagers — will also find Chinese exercise interesting and of value, especially when they take up programs which demand strenuous effort to strengthen their muscles. Needless to say, the representative or symbolic aspects of many of the exercises will attract both young and old.

With these considerations in mind, I thought it worthwhile to write a book

PREFACE

on Chinese exercise therapy for western readers, so that they might utilize this method of health care. As a physician trained in western medicine and with a research background in traditional Chinese medicine, I have been fortunate in being able to appreciate and evaluate traditional Chinese exercise therapy with an integrated point of view—from the standpoint of both western and Chinese medicine. The result is this practical guidebook on Chinese exercise therapy for the general reader and for people with chronic illness. In this book a number of traditional exercise programs are described in detail, and the application of these methods to a variety of diseases is dealt with in depth. Though Chinese methods are often used in conjunction with western methods in order to obtain the maximal therapeutic effect, this book emphasizes the Chinese methods.

The traditional system of Chinese exercise includes a strong preventive element for the promotion of general well-being and physical fitness. Regular and moderate exercise has long been considered valuable for health, fitness, and longevity. To reflect this tradition a number of well-known Chinese exercise programs are introduced in this book as examples of conditioning exercises. *Tai Chi*, *Yi Jin Jing*, and *Ba Duan Jin* all belong in this category. In addition, there are preventive health exercises specifically for sedentary people, the elderly, children, pregnant women, and athletes. In the sections for these programs, illustrations along with the description of the movements, as well as the benefits to be gained from the exercises, are presented. These exercises, many of which are characteristic of the traditional Chinese way, may be used to enhance physical strength, improve blood circulation, correct poor posture, increase flexibility and vigor, and to relax both body and mind. All will help promote the health of the exerciser.

The programs presented here are based on my own clinical experience and that of my colleagues in China. A substantial number of reports and presentations have demonstrated their usefulness and effectiveness in the management of disease. Chinese readers have shown much interest in these exercise programs, which I included in a Chinese text in 1976,* as have the many

---

*Zhuo Dahong: *Exercise Therapy in Chronic Diseases*. Beijing (Peking), People's Sports Press, 1976.

PREFACE

readers of the Japanese translation which followed. I shall be most happy if western readers also find this handbook useful in offering a simple and effective means to improve their health and fitness. It is also my sincere desire that this book will encourage the amalgamation of Chinese and western techniques of exercise therapy.

I am most indebted to my colleagues and associates at Zhongshan Medical College, Guangzhou (Canton), China, for their assistance in developing many of the programs presented in this book, to Dr. J. V. Basmajian of McMaster University and Dr. R. J. Shephard of the University of Toronto for their enthusiastic encouragement, to Dr. D. P. Barrett and Ms. S. W. Tauber for their valuable assistance in improving the style and language of the manuscript, to many other Canadian friends for their secretarial assistance, and to my publishers for their generous collaboration.

D. Zhuo
(Zhuo Dahong)
Guangzhou
The People's Republic of China, 1984

HOW TO USE THIS BOOK

This book contains a great variety of exercise programs for individuals with different levels of health and physical fitness, and for all age groups. Each program is designed to produce specific effects, so that choosing the programs appropriate for one's needs will be a simple matter.

Benefits of the various exercises

- Relaxing the mind and body, calming oneself, and developing a sense of confidence: *Chi Kung* and/or *Tai Chi Chuan,* and *Shier Duan Jin.*
- Promoting basic fitness: a combination of one of the Chinese traditional exercise programs and a preventive health exercise program designed for one of the following groups: athletes, children, the elderly, pregnant women, or the sedentary.
- Improving the health of the heart, blood vessels, and lungs: one of the preventive health exercise programs designed for the various groups, combined with brisk walking or jogging.
- Improving muscle tone, posture, and stance: *Ba Duan Jin* and *Yi Jin Jing.*
- Maintaining or improving flexibility of the joints and spine, preventing back and neck pain: a combination of a preventive health exercise program, *Yi Jin Jing* or *Tai Chi Chuan,* and *Shier Duan Jin.*

Note: To help control weight, jogging or brisk walking are recommended.

―――――――――――HOW TO USE THIS BOOK―――――――――――

For cure or better recovery from chronic disease, the third part of the book presents therapeutic exercise for particular diseases.

It is recommended that everyone using this book develop a daily exercise routine. Essential considerations in planning an exercise routine are the frequency, intensity, type, and time involved (FITT) in the exercises. If possible, the exercises should all be done in one or two daily sessions. Depending on individual needs, daily exercises should last at least ten minutes and may take up to half-an-hour. In most cases a moderate level of intensity is preferred. In terms of types of exercise, while the individual needs as described above should be considered, there is also room for personal preference.

For example, an exercise program for the average person is aimed at maintaining the health of the heart and lungs, increasing stamina, improving flexibility, and preventing mental stress. For these purposes, people in moderately good health may choose either of the following two programs.

(All exercises, except of course those for pregnant women, are suitable for both male and female exercisers.)

Example Program 1

Exercises for the sedentary, middle-aged, and those with mental stress

1. Preventive health exercise for the sedentary.
2. *Chi Kung for Fitness* (the Chinese way of meditation for mental and physical health).
3. *Shier Duan Jin* (which emphasizes self-massage or self-acupressure).

Note: It is preferable to practice these three sets of exercises together in one program.

Example Program 2

Exercises for the elderly and those with poor cardiovascular health or poor posture

1. *Ba Duan Jin* and/or *Yi Jin Jing*.
2. *Chi Kung for Relaxation*. (A relaxation-meditation technique.)
3. Brisk walking.
4. Preventive health exercise for the elderly.

Note: An elderly person should choose No. 4 (preventive health exercise for the elderly) instead of No. 1 (*Ba Duan Jin* and/or *Yi Jin Jing*).

PART I
Traditional Chinese Exercises

Introduction

Several basic exercise programs from the Chinese tradition are presented in this section. These popular and time-honored exercises are effective for both preventive and therapeutic purposes.

To obtain the maximum benefit from these exercises, one must try one's best to comply with certain requirements which are unique to the Chinese system of exercise.

In the first place, keep a peaceful mind and relaxed manner during the exercise. Focus your attention on the movement. You should be quite confident that you will benefit from doing the exercise.

Next, combine the movement with slow, gentle, and conscious breathing. This pattern of breathing will make you more relaxed and more aware of the movement.

Use your imagination when doing the exercise. Most of the traditional Chinese exercises, as indicated by their names, are representative or symbolic. Try to imagine what is suggested by the exercise, as if you were carrying out an imaginary task. For example, when doing the exercise "Shooting the eagle by drawing the bow with the hands," you should imagine there is an eagle in the sky and a bow in your hands. While watching the eagle attentively, you draw the bow to shoot the arrow at it.

Lastly, always combine exercise with self-administered massage. This is done either before exercise as a preparatory procedure, or following exercise to assist recovery and obtain benefits other than those directly resulting from the exercise. For example, massage on the face and neck produces tranquilizing effects and helps concentrate the mind on preparing for the exercises; massage on the joints following exercises induces a sense of relaxation and ease around the joints. In addition, massage on acupuncture points results in effects specific to those points as described in the following sections of this book.

For indications to a particular exercise, one may refer to the text of that section as well as the following sections dealing with particular diseases.

It is advisable to adhere to a set of programs which you find to suit you best. It is also acceptable to combine several programs at one time, or to alternate different programs from time to time.

CHAPTER I

Tai Chi Chuan

Translated literally the Chinese word *Tai* means great, *Chi* means origin, and *Chuan*, exercise with the hands. Hence *Tai Chi Chuan* is an exercise of great origin using the hands. It is so named because *Tai Chi* is regarded as the mother of *Yin* and *Yang,* while *Yin* and *Yang* are regarded as the parents of all things.* A good balance between *Yin* and *Yang* is essential to health, and *Tai Chi Chuan* is so valuable because it incorporates *Yin* and *Yang* in a balanced manner.

Tai Chi is a gentle and relaxing form of exercise. My research during my stay at the University of Toronto established that the average energy cost for the long form of *Tai Chi Chuan* is equal to walking at the speed of approximately 3½ miles per hour, putting it in the category of moderate exercise.

In my own experience and that of other Chinese physicians, *Tai Chi Chuan* produces remarkable effects in the treatment of a number of illnesses. It is also of great benefit to people in a variety of age groups, and with varying constitutions and levels of health. For those with emotional problems or prone to mental stress, *Tai Chi* brings relaxation and modification of the psychological profile, developing better concentration, attention, composure, self-confidence, and self-control.

For people with hypertension, it is a natural way to lower blood pressure. This effect occurs either immediately after a practice session or after a long-

---

* *Yin* and *Yang* are the two universal energies, which are polarized, and contain and complement each other. *Yang* is the creative initiator, and *Yin,* the cooperative, receptive energy.

term period of training. In turn, symptoms such as headache, dizziness, and insomnia are relieved.

For those with mild arthritis or rheumatism, practicing *Tai Chi* will increase the flexibility of the joints and prevent restriction of movement.

For people with atherosclerosis, it helps improve the circulation in the hands, legs, and feet. Symptoms such as numbness and weakness of the hands and feet will be relieved.

Derived from *Tao Yin* (the Way of Yin), *Tai Chi Chuan* has absorbed all the best qualities of Chinese traditional therapeutic exercises. As the movements are gentle and slow, they are particularly suitable for the middle-aged and elderly. Performance of *Tai Chi* requires relaxation of the muscles of the wrists, arms, shoulders, chest, abdomen, and back. The gentleness of the movement enables the performer to experience a feeling of relaxation, comfort, and ease. It may be said that *Tai Chi Chuan* brings peacefulness and rest to the mind. Meanwhile, relaxation of the muscles leads to relaxation of the arterioles, in turn reducing blood pressure. This is why a hypertensive patient may benefit from *Tai Chi*.

Tai Chi movements are directed by thought rather than by strength. While performing them, one must be relaxed and quiet, with the attention directed towards each movement of the exercise. Such concentration will bring relief in cases with emotional disorders, and provides an excellent exercise for the mind.

Tai Chi Chuan involves all the muscles and joints of the limbs and trunk. Each and every movement involves all muscles of the body. It is also a breathing exercise. During the practice of *Tai Chi,* breathing should be deep, steady, rhythmic, and gentle. Inhalation and exhalation should coincide with certain movements and in accordance with a set routine.

With the lumbar region as the axis of its movement, *Tai Chi Chuan* involves exercise of the trunk and facilitates the circulation of blood in the abdomen, thus improving digestion.

The intensity of *Tai Chi* is relatively low compared to jogging and other sports. Taking Simplified *Tai Chi Chuan* as an example, investigations have determined changes in physical functions during or immediately after the performance of these movements to be very slight (the heart rate measured at

Tai Chi Chuan

105 beats per minute; blood pressure, 128/70 mmHg; pulmonary ventilation, 8.54 liters per minute; and energy cost, 2.3581 kcal per minute — only 11.92 kcal is expended if the exercise is completed in five minutes). The intensity of the older form of *Tai Chi* is a little higher than that of Simplified *Tai Chi Chuan*, but is still fairly low. Because of this low intensity, *Tai Chi* generally does not lead to fatigue or stress.

In addition to all its other benefits, and due to the complexity of its movements, *Tai Chi Chuan* helps improve coordination and balance.

Because of all this, *Tai Chi* has enjoyed much popularity among the Chinese people for over six hundred years, and is still highly valued today.

How to practice *Tai Chi* correctly

To obtain the maximum therapeutic effect of *Tai Chi Chuan*, one must practice it in accordance with certain principles:

- All movement should be gentle and soft, with the breath smooth and natural. *Tai Chi* should be performed gently, lightly, and in slow progression. Take your steps as lightly as a cat walks. Stretch your arms as gently as if you were pulling a thread of silk. It is desirable to move very slowly so that it takes 5–9 minutes to finish a set of Simplified *Tai Chi Chuan*.
- While performing *Tai Chi*, practice diaphragmatic breathing (abdominal breathing) naturally and rhythmically. Breathe in when doing raising or stretching movements; breathe out when doing lowering or bending movements. Never hold your breath during its performance.
- Relax the body and take an easy and comfortable stance. *Tai Chi Chuan* abhors straining and "grunting" motions. The stance should be easy and composed, and the body should be relaxed, especially the lower back and abdomen. It is inappropriate to strain the chest. Relax the muscles of the back so that the shoulders are dropped and relaxed. Your posture should follow these basic guidelines: Hold your chest in and straighten your back; drop your shoulders and lower your elbows. Then your stance will be easy and comfortable and your body will maintain good posture.
- Direct every movement with close attention, but do the exercises as effortlessly as possible. During the performance of *Tai Chi*, it is important to

allow your every movement to be directed consciously. You should have the image of the movement in your mind. Meditate over it quietly. "Draw" the image of the movement in your mind at the same time as you actually draw the image of the movement with your arms and legs.
- The strength of your muscles should be so controlled that you are making no visible effort, nor straining. Your limbs should move effortlessly, though actually you are using some strength to accomplish this.

It must be emphasized that *Tai Chi Chuan* is a very complicated exercise and cannot be self-taught. One must learn it from an experienced teacher. Fortunately, there are many *Tai Chi* centers in North America, and competent teachers are available in many cities. The following guidelines may be useful to those who are looking for a teacher of *Tai Chi*.
- Try to find a teacher who has been practicing *Tai Chi* for more than five years and has had experience in teaching it.
- If possible, select a teacher from among the active members of a well-established *Tai Chi* society.
- A *Tai Chi* teacher with a background of training in physical health education, or in health and life sciences, is preferred. Also, it is better to choose a health-oriented instructor than one oriented towards martial arts. However, proficiency in skill and knowledge should be the top criterion in making the choice.
- National origin is not important in selecting a *Tai Chi* teacher. Very often Caucasian teachers are as competent as their Chinese counterparts in teaching *Tai Chi*. For teachers of any nationality, an interest in and understanding of the Chinese philosophy of health and exercise is a definite asset to their teaching.

Simplified *Tai Chi Chuan*

Commencing form (1-4)

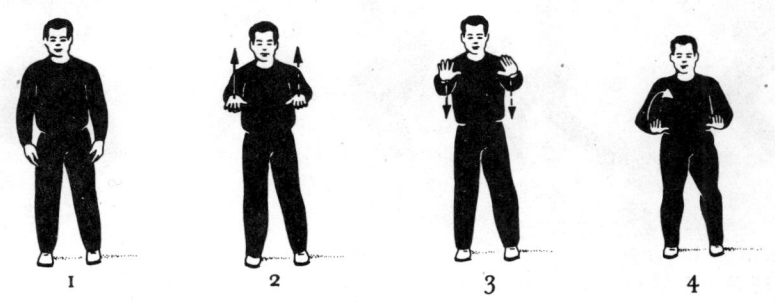

1 2 3 4

Parting the wild horse's mane on the left side (5-9)

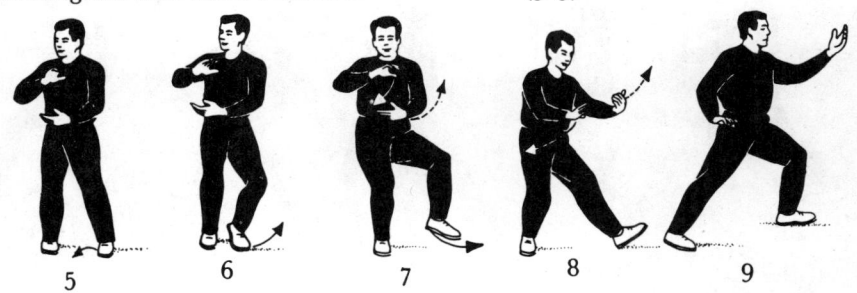

5 6 7 8 9

Parting the wild horse's mane on the right side (10-14)

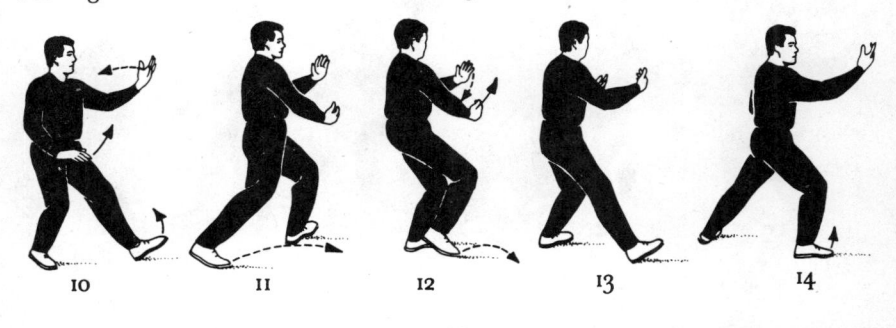

10 11 12 13 14

TRADITIONAL CHINESE EXERCISES

Parting the wild horse's mane on the left side (15-19)

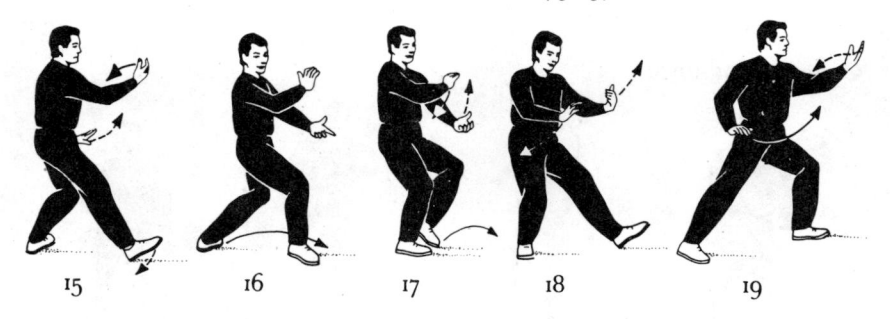

The white crane spreads its wings (20-22)

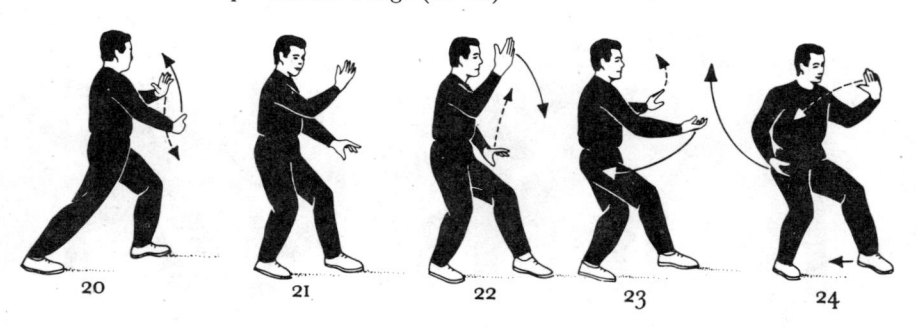

Brush knee and twist step on the left side (23-29)

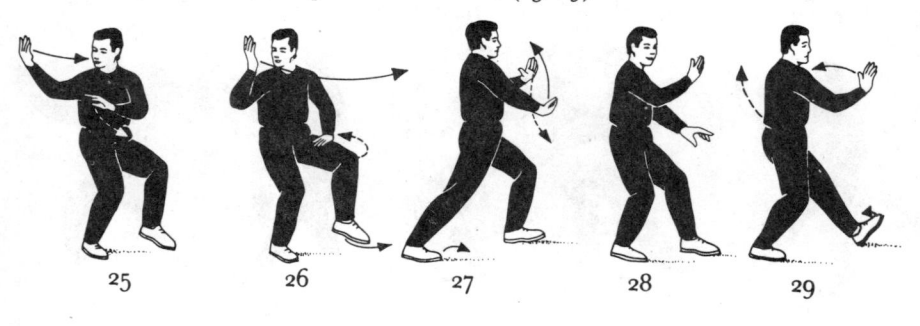

Tai Chi Chuan

Brush knee and twist step on the right side (30-34)

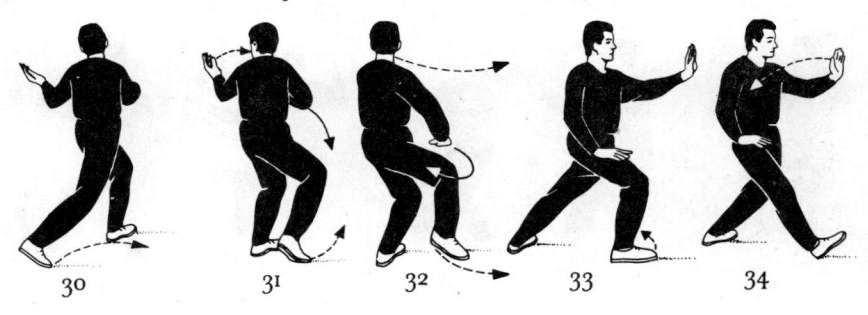

30   31   32   33   34

Brush knee and twist step on the left side (35-38)

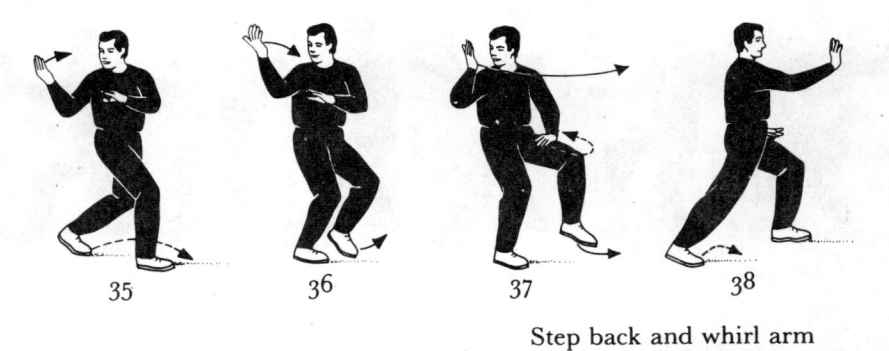

35   36   37   38

The hand strums the lute (39-41)

Step back and whirl arm on the left side (42-45)

39   40   41   42   43

TRADITIONAL CHINESE EXERCISES

Step back and whirl arm on the right side (46–48)

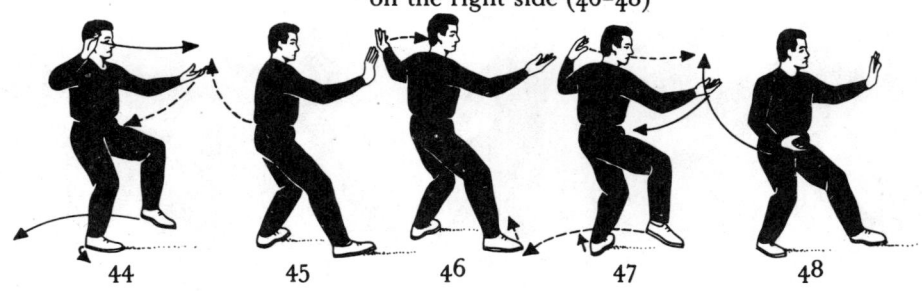

44 45 46 47 48

Step back and whirl arm on the left side (49–51)

Step back and whirl arm on the right side (52–54)

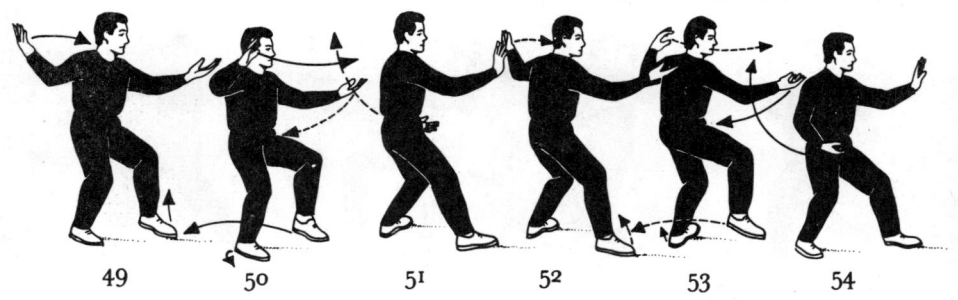

49 50 51 52 53 54

Grasp the bird's tail — left style (55–66)

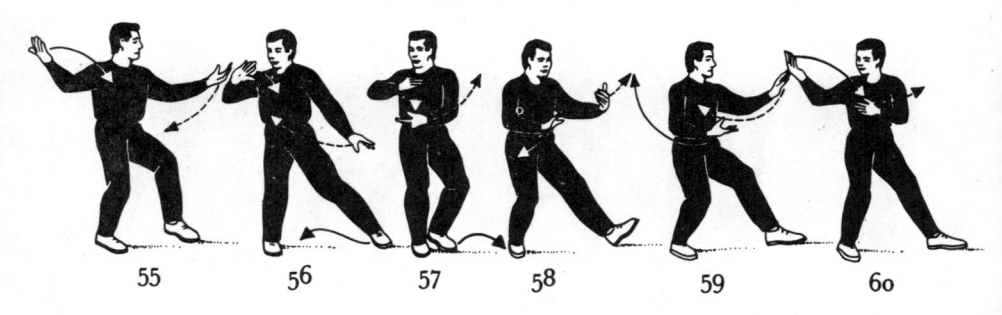

55 56 57 58 59 60

Tai Chi Chuan

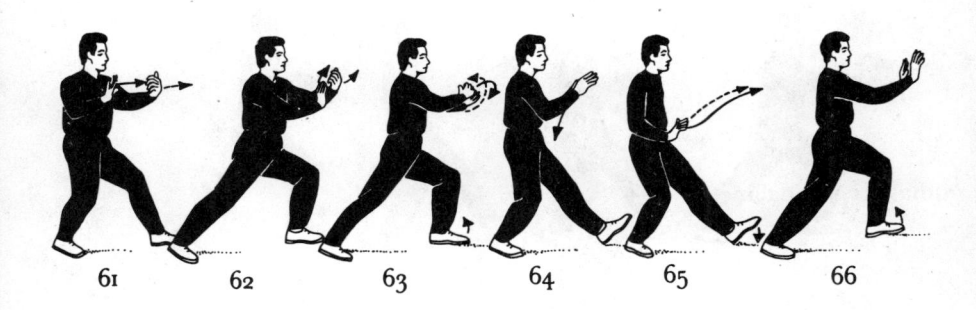

Grasp the bird's tail — right style (67–80)

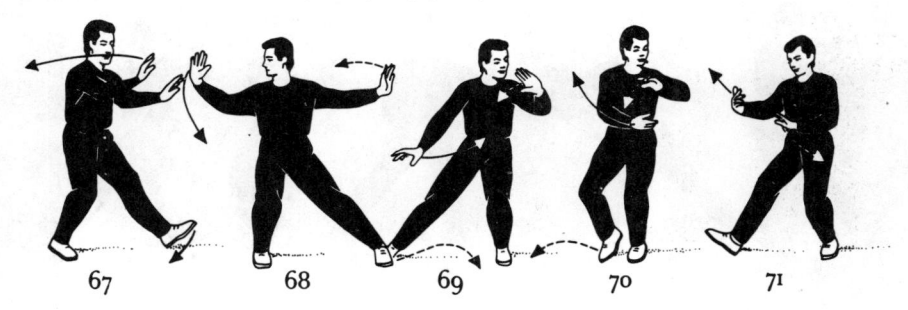

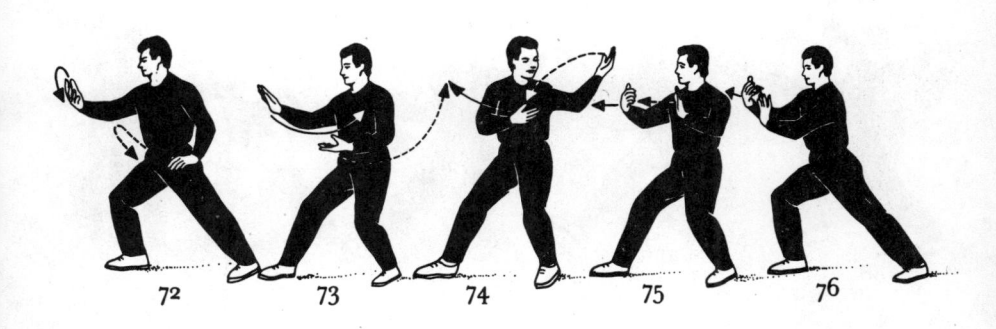

TRADITIONAL CHINESE EXERCISES

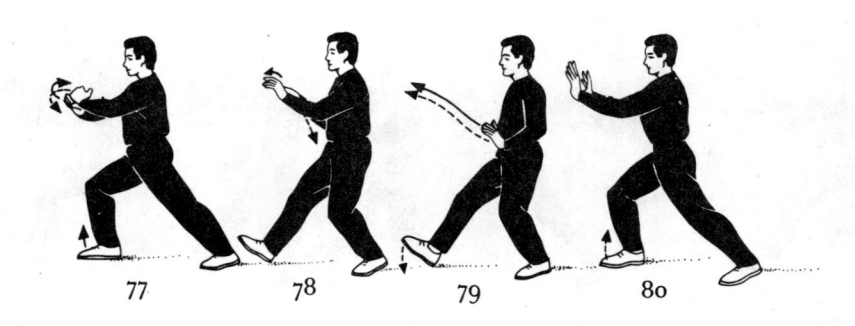

77 78 79 80

Single whip (81–86)

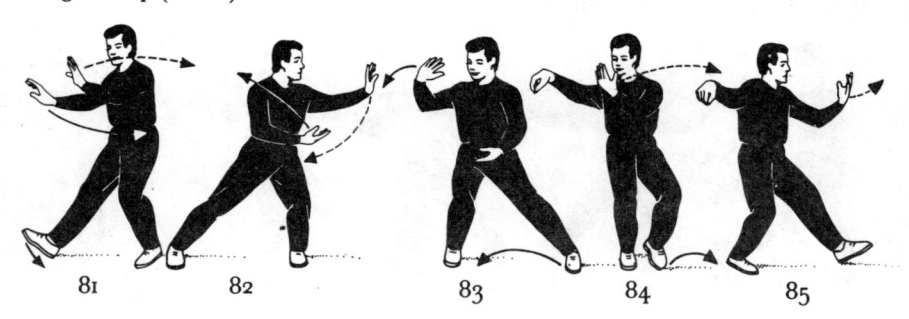

81 82 83 84 85

Wave the hands like clouds (87–100)

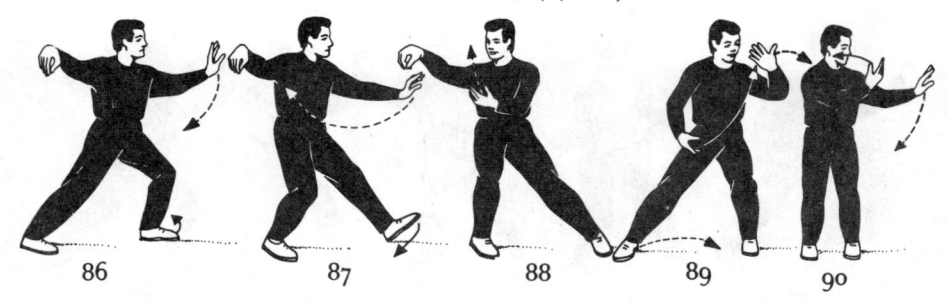

86 87 88 89 90

28

Tai Chi Chuan

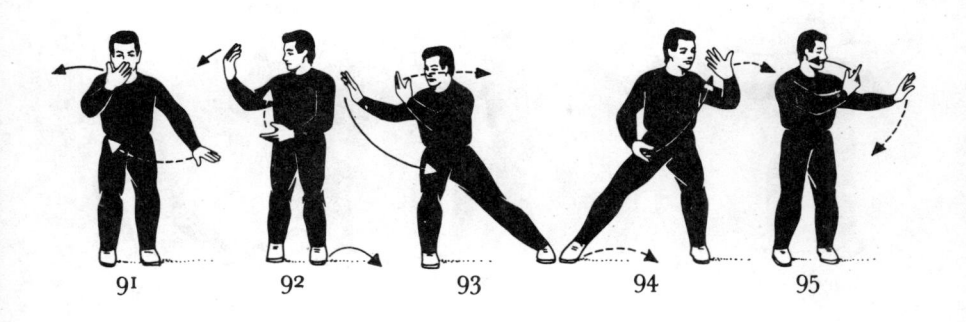

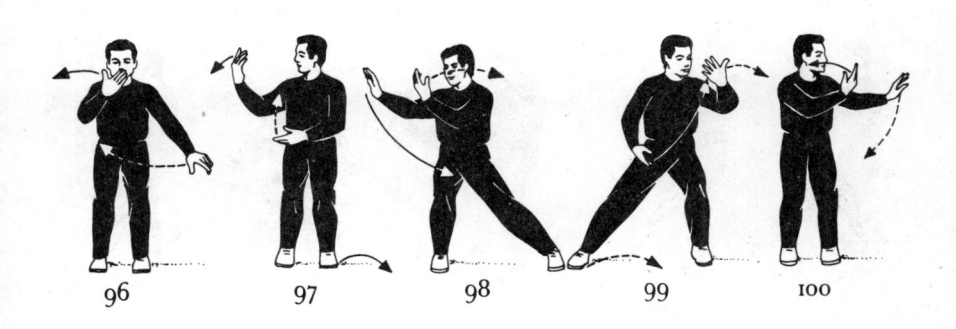

91 92 93 94 95

96 97 98 99 100

Single whip (101-5)

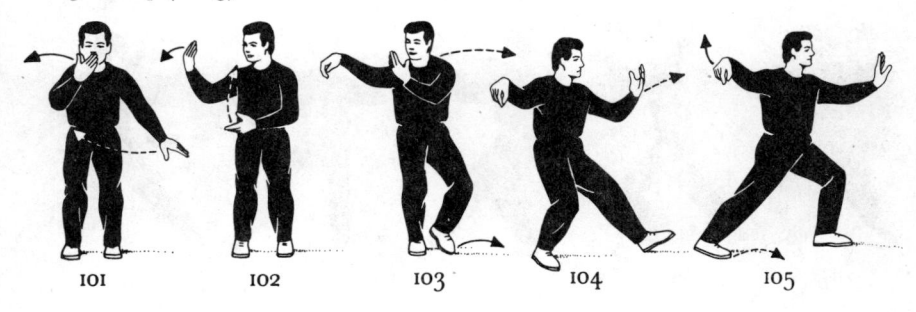

101 102 103 104 105

TRADITIONAL CHINESE EXERCISES

Pat the horse high (106-7)   **Kick with the right heel (108-13)**

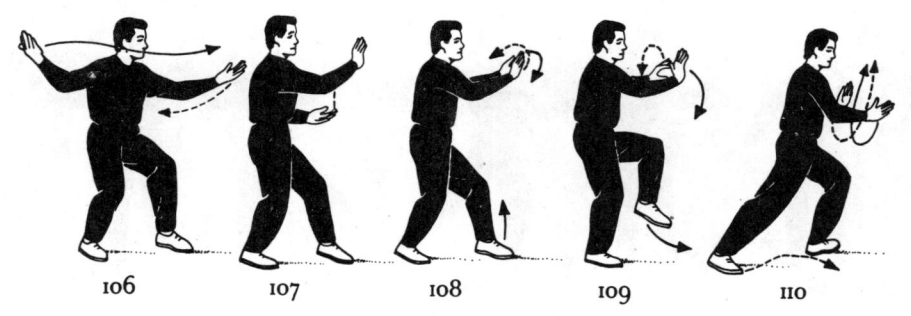

106   107   108   109   110

Strike opponent's ears with both fists (114-17)

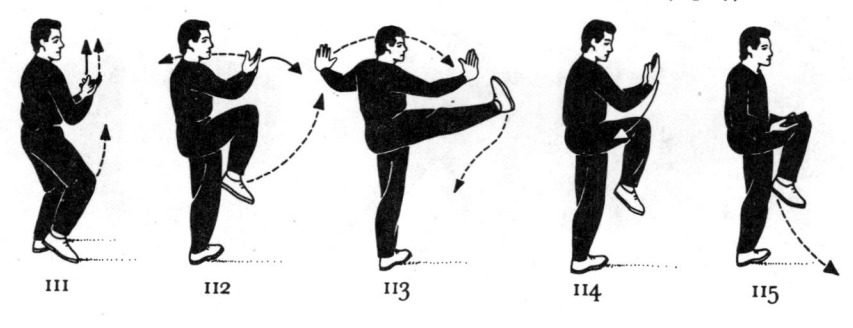

111   112   113   114   115

Turn and kick with the left heel (118-23)

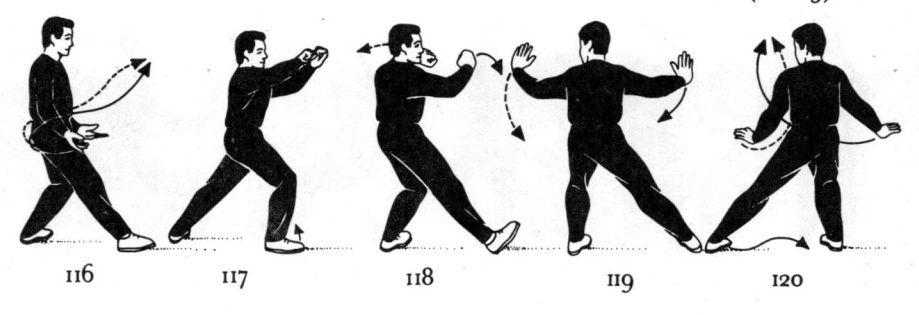

116   117   118   119   120

Tai Chi Chuan

Push down and stand on one leg — left style (124-30)

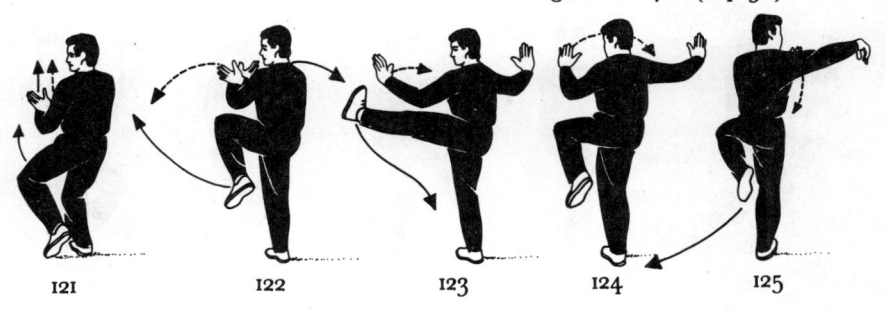

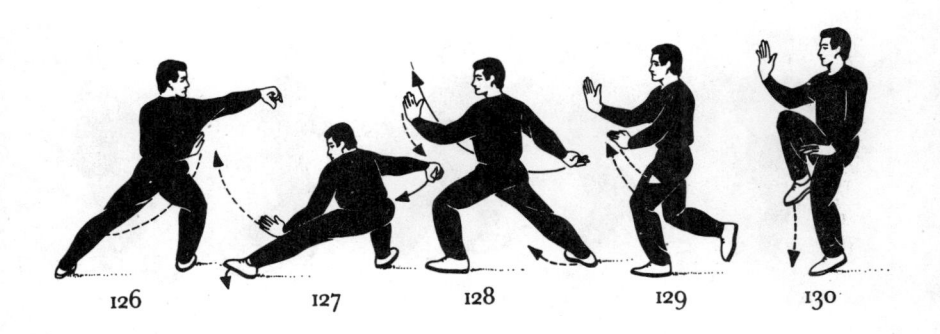

121　122　123　124　125

126　127　128　129　130

Push down and stand on one leg — right style (131-37)

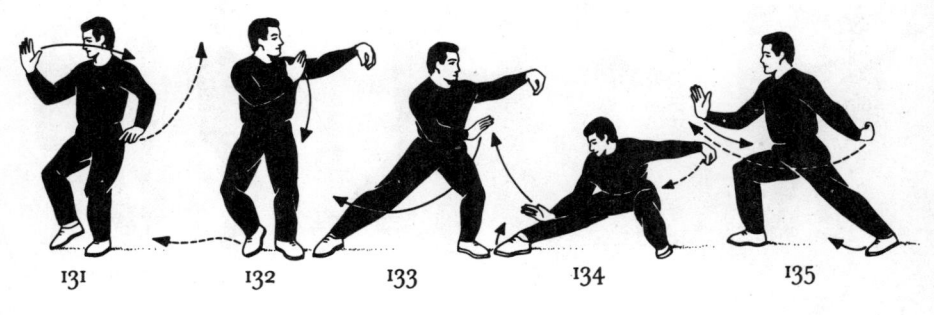

131　132　133　134　135

31

TRADITIONAL CHINESE EXERCISES

Work at shuttles — left style (138–42)

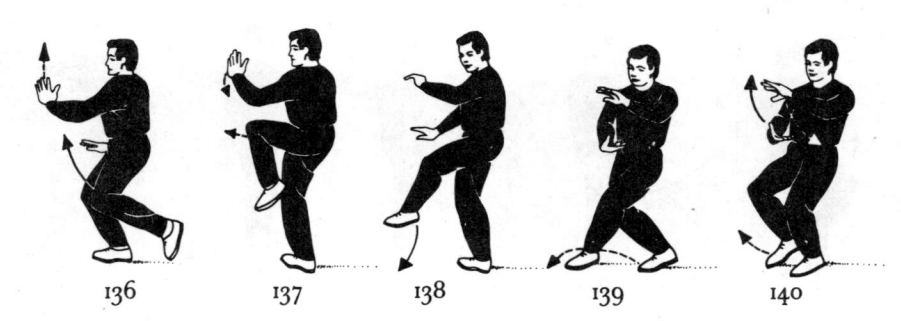

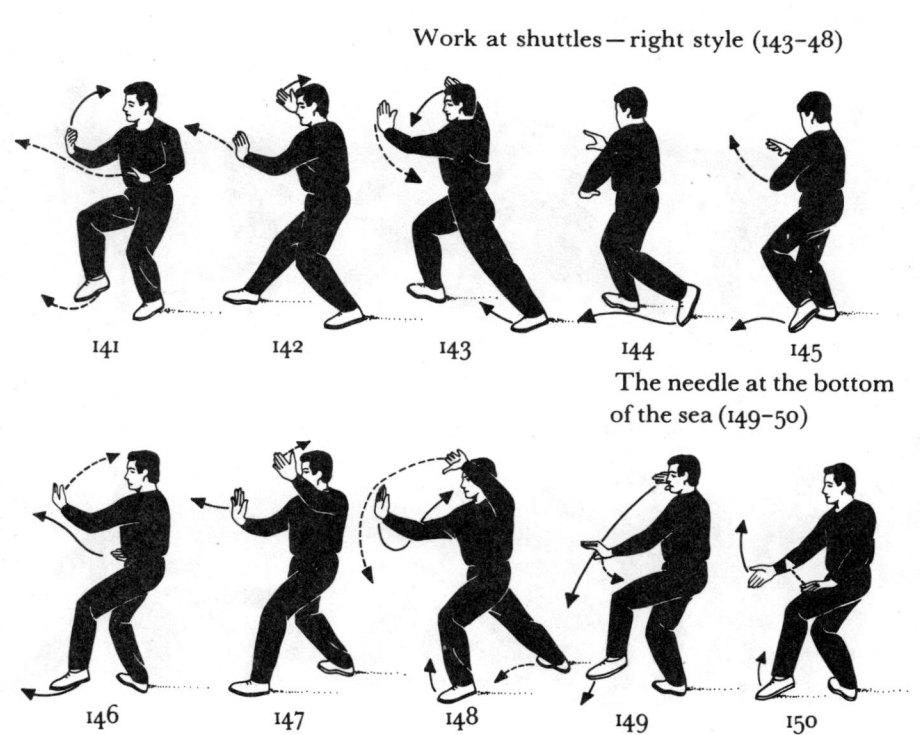

136   137   138   139   140

Work at shuttles — right style (143–48)

141   142   143   144   145

The needle at the bottom of the sea (149–50)

146   147   148   149   150

Tai Chi Chuan

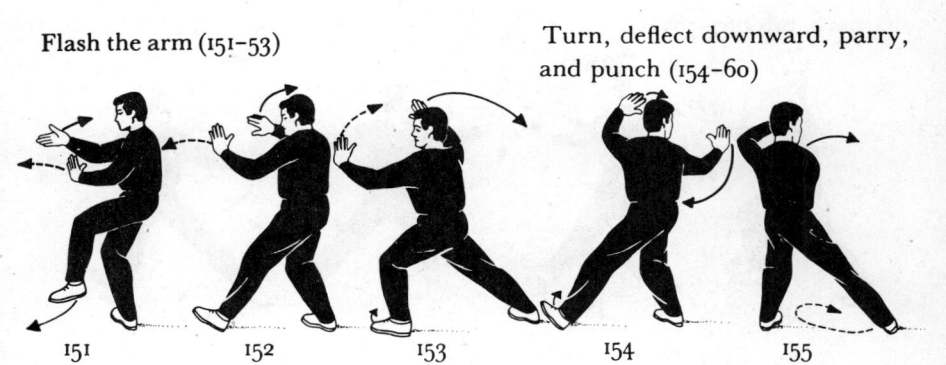

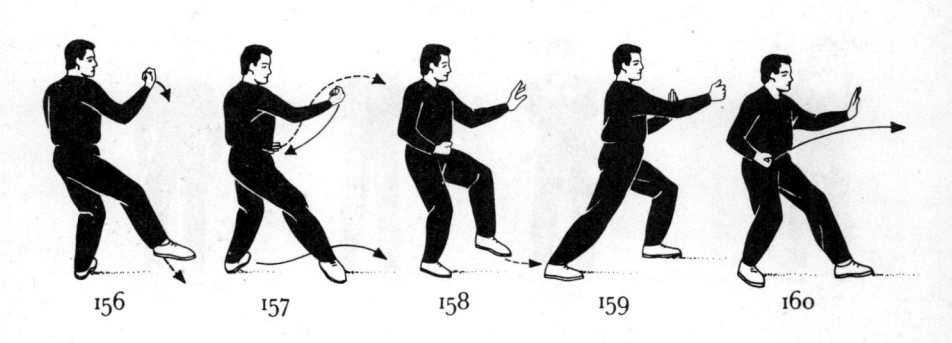

Flash the arm (151-53)

Turn, deflect downward, parry, and punch (154-60)

151 152 153 154 155 156 157 158 159 160

Apparent close-up (161-66)

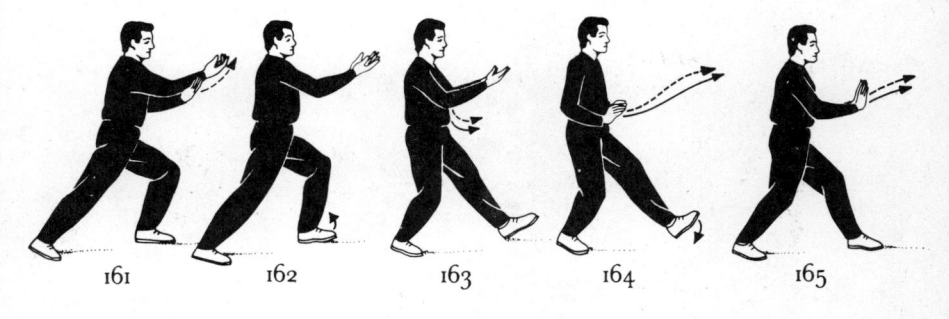

161 162 163 164 165

TRADITIONAL CHINESE EXERCISES

Cross hands (167–70)

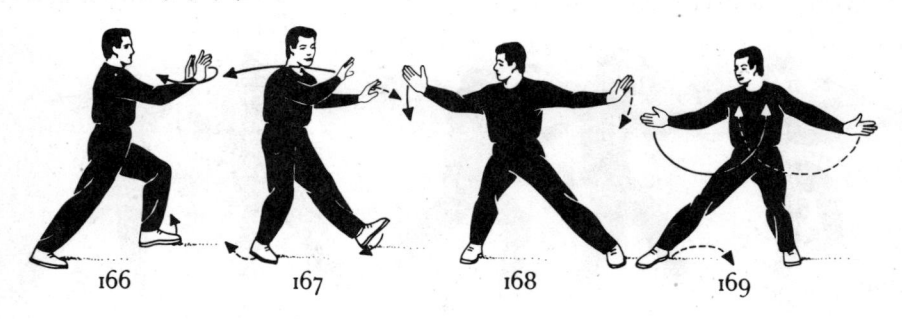

166   167   168   169

Closing form (171–73)

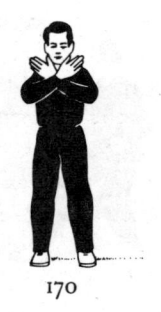

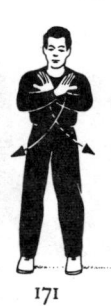

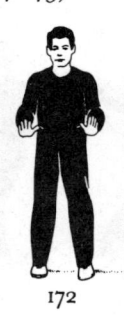

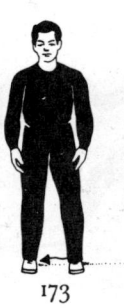

170   171   172   173

CHAPTER II

Yi Jin Jing — Muscle Strengthening Exercises

Yi Jin Jing is one of China's traditional forms of calisthenics. Its origin may be traced back over a thousand years. It consists of twelve exercises involving the head, arms, and trunk, and is performed in a standing position. Essentially, this program of exercise is isometric in nature. Unlike *Tai Chi Chuan,* Yi *Jin Jing* movements should be performed with significant vigor, though the motions are slow and appear gentle. Along with the vigorous movement, there should be relative stillness of mind, with the attention focusing on various parts of the body. As an exercise effective in strengthening muscles, it is still widely practiced today by Chinese masseurs and traditional bone surgeons, as well as by the average person wishing to maintain good muscle tone.

Yi Jin Jing can be done in full sequence or selectively. When done in full, as in the case of fitness training for younger people, one begins with Exercise 1 and proceeds in a smooth succession until the last exercise (Number 12) is completed. When done selectively, the exercises can be chosen in accordance with the needs of the exerciser. For example, those with neck pain will choose Exercise 4 (Reaching the stars) and Exercise 7 (Pulling the ear). To improve posture, Exercises 1, 2, and 3 can be chosen, while Exercise 8 is best for developing the knees and thighs. Individuals with hypertension should not do Exercises 10, 11, or 12, so as to prevent the risk of getting a headache or aggravating an already existing headache when lowering the head. The twelve exercises of *Yi Jin Jing* are as follows:

TRADITIONAL CHINESE EXERCISES

Exercises 1 thru 3 are stretching exercises, good for improving posture and expanding the chest. Like the other exercises (Numbers 4 thru 12) of *Yi Jin Jing,* they are called body/mind exercises, since attention and imagery are emphasized, helping to cultivate an alert mind. These three should be performed once each and in succession.

EXERCISE 1: *Making a gesture of respect with both hands facing the chest.*

STARTING POSITION: Standing, arms at sides, feet apart shoulder width, back erect, eyes straight ahead.
MOVEMENT: 1. Raise the arms slowly from the sides until they reach a horizontal position, palms downward, elbows straight. 2. Turn the palms inward, bend the elbows to let the hands approach the chest and stop at a distance of 6 inches (15 cm) in front of the chest.

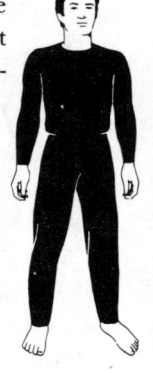

STARTING POSITION

Note: This exercise, as an initial and preparatory step, serves to adjust the body (relaxed and comfortable), adjust the mind (peaceful and concentrated), and adjust the breathing (smooth and natural).

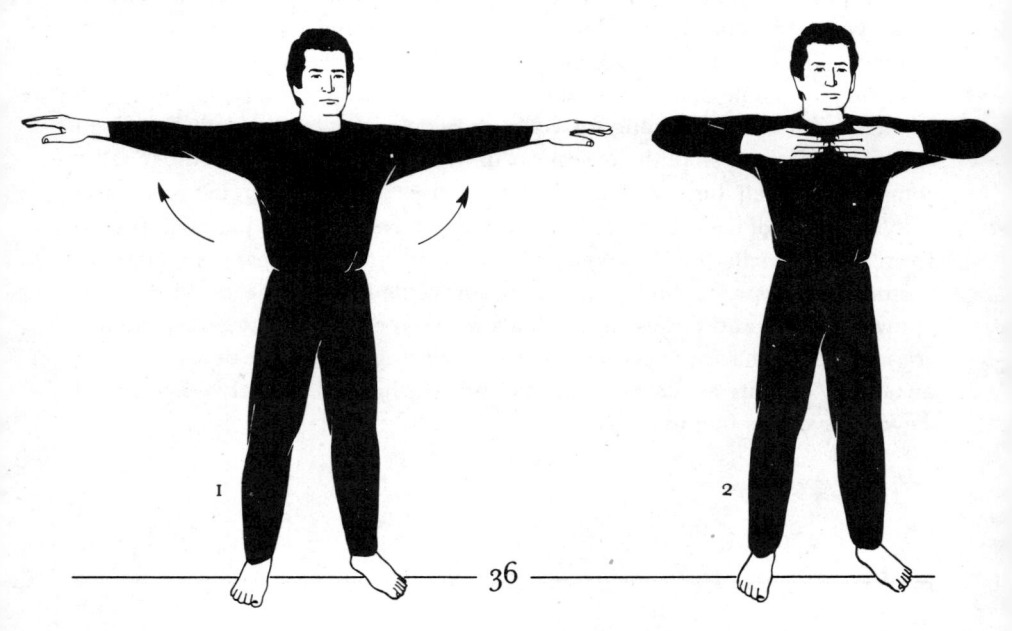

Yi Jin Jing — *Muscle Strengthening Exercises*

EXERCISE 2: *Heaving.*

STARTING POSITION: Standing, feet apart shoulder width, arms at sides, back erect, eyes straight ahead.
MOVEMENT: 1. Toes firmly touching the ground, turn the palms upward. 2. Raise the heels slightly about one inch (2–3 cm). Toes touching the ground, extend the arms horizontally, palms upward, and hold. Attention is focused on palms and toes. Breathe naturally.

Note: Movements of hands and feet should be performed simultaneously.

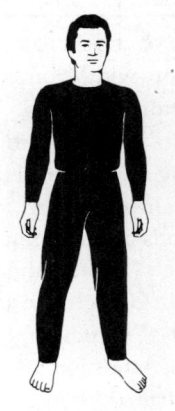

STARTING POSITION

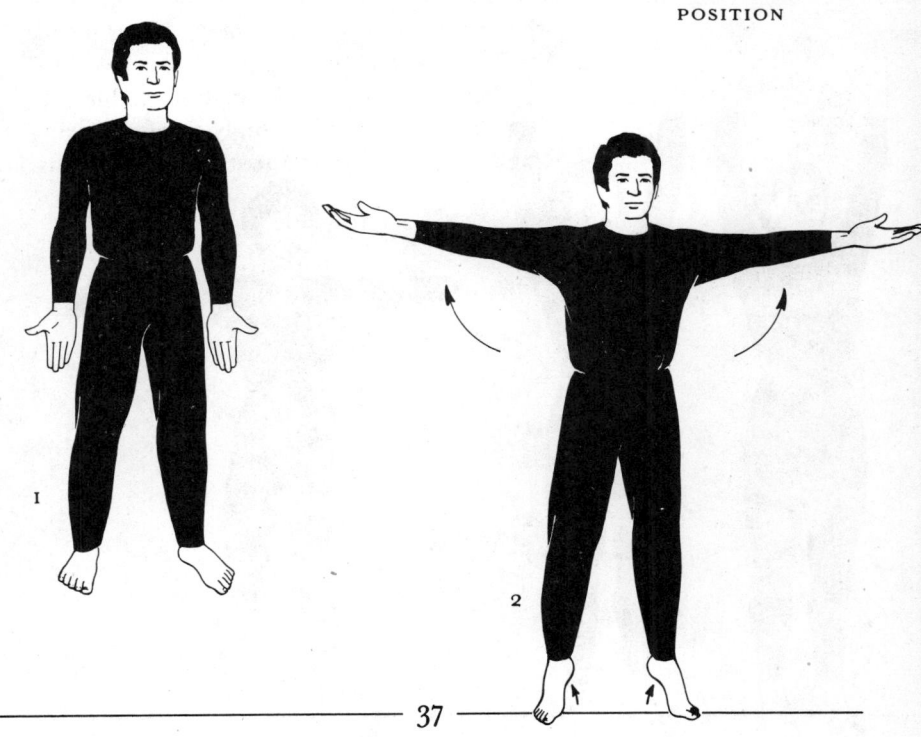

TRADITIONAL CHINESE EXERCISES

EXERCISE 3: *Pushing towards the sky.*

STARTING POSITION: Standing, feet apart shoulder width, arms extended horizontally, palms upward.

MOVEMENT: 1. Raise the arms slowly from the side, as if drawing an arc, until they reach a vertical position. 2. Then turn palms upward, fingers pointing inward as though the hands are pushing up towards the sky. Meanwhile raise the heels higher than in Exercise 2, toes touching the ground. Clench the jaw and place the tip of the tongue against the roof of the mouth, breathing smoothly and deeply. Attention is focused on both palms (watching the palms from the mind). 3. Clench the fists and slowly lower the arms to the "heaving" position (arms extended horizontally out to the sides, with the palms open and upward). Heels down.

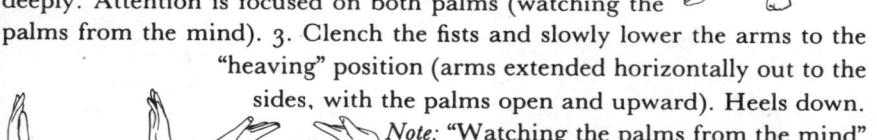

Note: "Watching the palms from the mind" does not mean looking at the palms with the eyes. It simply means focusing your attention on the palms.

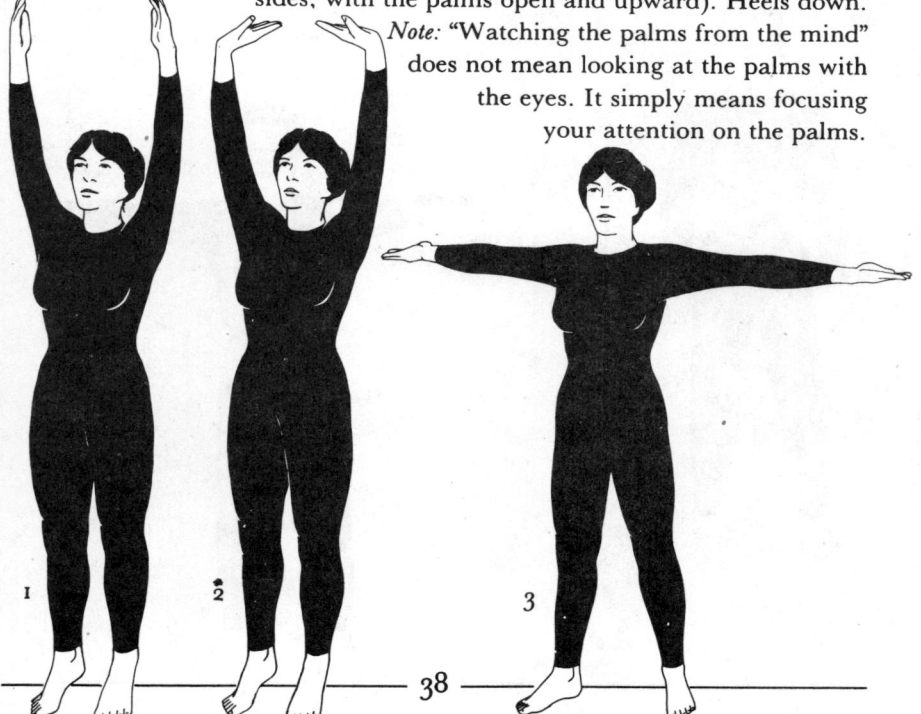

Yi Jin Jing — *Muscle Strengthening Exercises*

EXERCISE 4: *Reaching the stars.*

This exercise develops flexibility of the shoulder joints and the upper spine. It helps to prevent the frozen shoulders and stiff neck common among the middle-aged and elderly. Since the exercise involves static contraction of the arm muscles while holding the reaching position, it is also good for strengthening the arms.

STARTING POSITION: Standing, feet apart shoulder width, arms extended horizontally, palms open and upward.

MOVEMENT: 1. Raise the right arm slowly until it reaches a vertical position. Turn the palm downward, fingers together pointing inward. Raise the head upward and turn right, with the eyes looking at the right palm. Meanwhile, bring the left arm down and turn the left palm with the back of the hand touching the back. Hold this position for a while. Take 3–5 breaths. 2. Raise the left arm (as in step 1 for the right arm). Raise the head and turn left with the eyes looking at the left palm. Bring the right arm down and touch the back with the back of the right hand. Hold. Take 3–5 breaths.

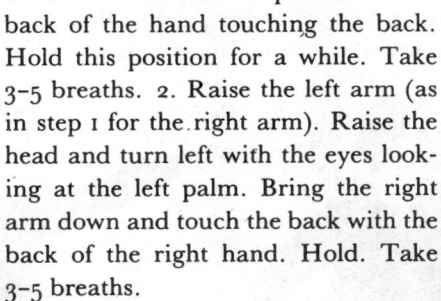

Repeat this exercise 3–5 times.

Note: While looking at the upper hand, attention is focused on the back, which is being touched by the other hand. When breathing in, press the back lightly with the hand. When breathing out, relax. Breathing should be rythmic, smooth, and slow.

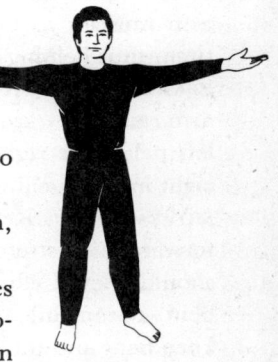

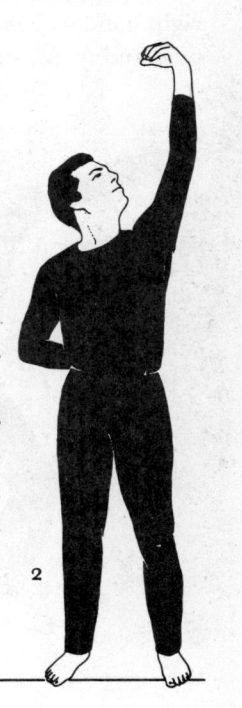

STARTING POSITION

1

2

39

TRADITIONAL CHINESE EXERCISES

EXERCISE 5: *Pulling the tails of nine oxen.*

This is an isometric exercise which involves contracting the arm muscles as tightly as possible for the required length of time, thus helping develop strength in the arms.

STARTING POSITION: Standing, feet apart shoulder width, left arm raised upward, the head turned up with eyes looking at the left palm, the right arm flexed backward with the back of the right hand touching the lower back.

MOVEMENT: 1. Remove the right hand from the back. Bring it forward and stretch the arm until the hand is raised to the shoulder level, elbow slightly bent, fingers together and slightly bent. Meanwhile, the right foot takes a step forward with the knee bent and the left leg stretching straight behind. Bring the left arm down and stretch it behind, fingers together and slightly bent, palms upward. Breathe in, and focus attention on the right hand which is pulling with effort, as if pulling the tails of oxen. Breathe out, and focus attention on the left hand which is now pulling with similar

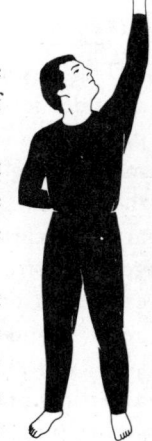

STARTING POSITION

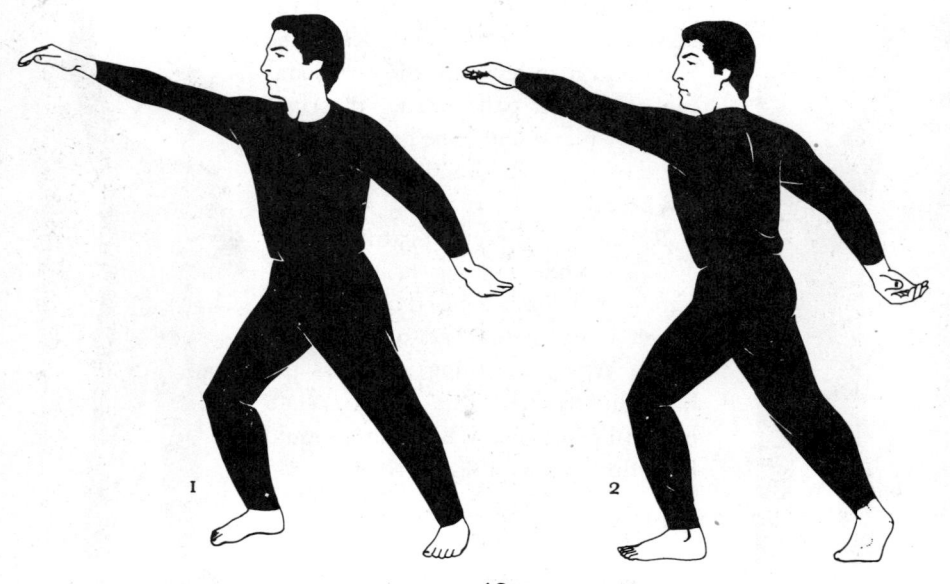

40

Yi Jin Jing — *Muscle Strengthening Exercises*

effort from behind, as if pulling the tails of oxen. Repeat several times. As a result of straining, the legs, trunk, shoulders and elbows will tremble slightly when pulling. 2. The left foot takes a step forward with the knee bent and the right leg stretching straight behind. Turn the left wrist and stretch the left arm forward. Bring the right arm down and stretch it behind (same position as step 1, only reversed). Breathe in, and focus attention on the left hand. Breathe out, focusing attention on the right hand. The requirements for the pulling movement are the same as in step 2.

Repeat this exercise 3-5 times.

Note: Breathe naturally with the abdomen relaxed. The pulling should be somewhat strained.

EXERCISE 6: *Pushing the mountain.*

This exercise strengthens the arms and helps correct a rounded upper back.

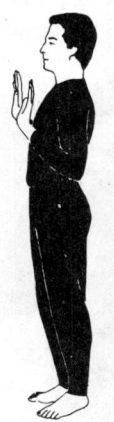

STARTING POSITION: Standing, feet together, elbows bent at sides with fingers spread and pointing upward, palms forward.

MOVEMENT: Hands erect and form a right angle at the wrists, palms outward ("mountain pushing hands"). Push hands slowly forward, increasing the effort gradually until the elbows are fully extended. Meanwhile keep the body straight, eyes straight forward. Then bring the hands back to the starting position alongside the chest.

STARTING POSITION

Repeat this exercise 3-5 times.

Note: At the end of the pushing, effort is exerted to the maximum, as if you are pushing a mountain. Breathe out while pushing. Breathe in when relaxing.

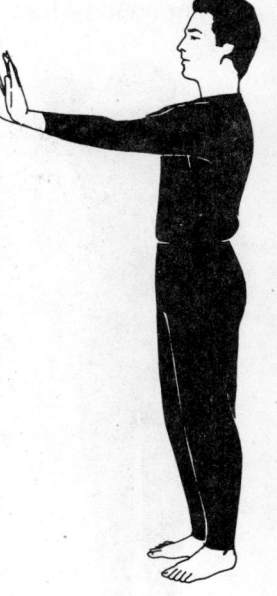

TRADITIONAL CHINESE EXERCISES

EXERCISE 7: *Pulling the ear.*

The benefits gained from this exercise are much the same as those in Exercise 4 (Reaching the stars), though to a lesser extent.

STARTING POSITION: Reach standing: Standing, feet together, arms fully extended forward horizontally, palms facing forward.

MOVEMENT: 1. Raise the right hand to the back of the head. Press the head with the palm, and pull and press the left ear with fingers. The right shoulder is fully extended. Meanwhile, turn the head to the left and place the left hand on the back with the back of the hand touching the space between the shoulder blades. Breathe in, pulling and pressing the left ear with the right hand. At this time, there will be a sense of strain at the head and right elbow. Attention is focused on the right elbow. Breathe out and relax. Repeat the above breathing 3-5 times. 2. Bring the right hand down and put it on the back with the back of the hand touching the space between the shoulder blades. Raise the left hand to the back of the head. Press the head with the palm, pull and press the right ear with the fingers, lightly. The left shoulder is fully extended. Meanwhile, turn the head to the right. Breathe in, pulling and pressing the right ear with the left hand. At this time, the head and elbow again experience a sense of strain. Attention is focused on the left elbow. Breathe out and relax. Repeat this 3-5 times.

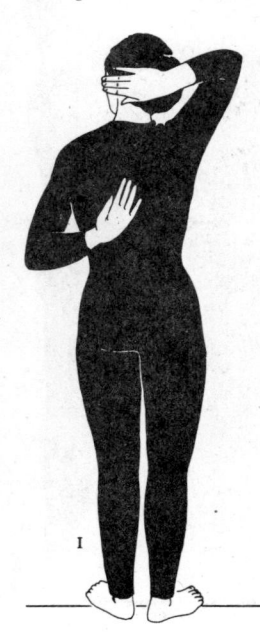

Repeat the entire exercise 3-5 times.

Note: Keep the body straight and the breathing smooth.

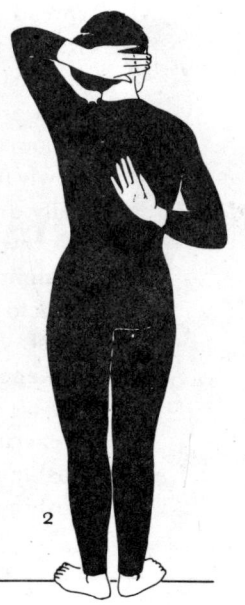

Yi Jin Jing—*Muscle Strengthening Exercises*

EXERCISE 8: *Lifting the plates.*

This is a good exercise for strengthening the thighs and knees. It is recommended for both prevention and treatment of weak and painful knees resulting from the degeneration of their cartilage.

STARTING POSITION: Standing, feet apart shoulder width, arms extended sidewards at shoulder level, palms downward.

MOVEMENT: 1. Bend the knees (ride standing), head and back remaining straight. Bend the elbows and press the hands downward with increasing effort as the knees continue gradually to bend, fingers apart with the thumbs pointing inward. Press the hands down to about 6-8 inches (15-20 cm) above the knees. 2. Turn the palms upward. Raise the hands slowly as if you were lifting heavy objects weighing a thousand pounds, and begin straightening the knees gradually to a standing position.

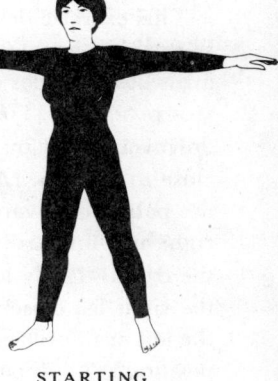

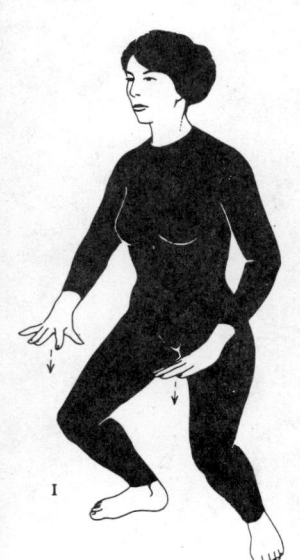

STARTING POSITION

Repeat this exercise 3-5 times.

Note: The movement should be slow. Strenuous effort must be made in doing the "lifting." During the exercise, close the mouth and place the tip of the tongue against the roof of the mouth, eyes wide open and straight ahead. Breathe out as the hands press down, breathe in as they lift up.

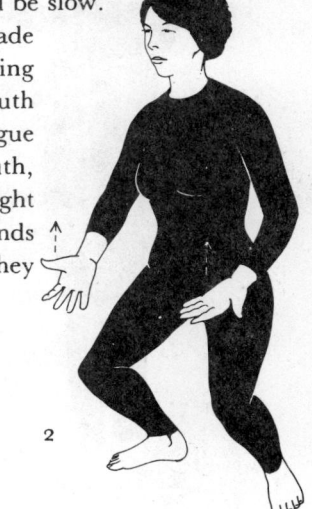

1

2

43

TRADITIONAL CHINESE EXERCISES

EXERCISE 9: *Stretching the arms.*

This exercise develops the arms.
STARTING POSITION: Standing, feet slightly apart, arms bent at sides of chest, palms up.
MOVEMENT: 1. Turn the left hand with the palm downward and make a loose fist. Bring the left hand close to the hip. Meanwhile, turn the right hand with the palm downward and make a loose fist. Stretch the right arm forward towards the left. Turn the head and the trunk slightly to the left at the same time. 2. Bring the right fist close to the right hip. Meanwhile stretch the left arm forward towards the right (to the reverse of position 1). Repeat 3–5 times.

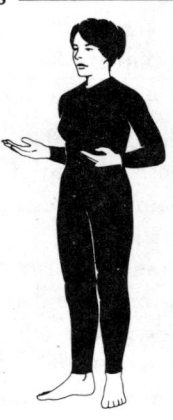

STARTING POSITION

Note: Breathe in through the nose when stretching the arm. Breathe out through the mouth when the stretching is completed.

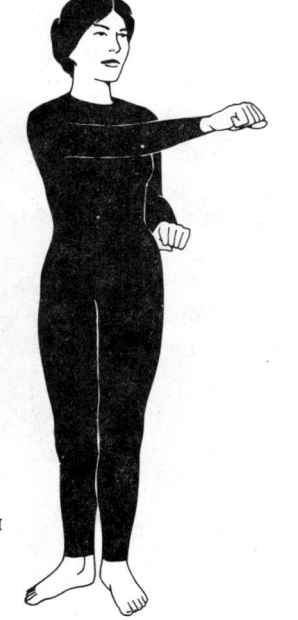

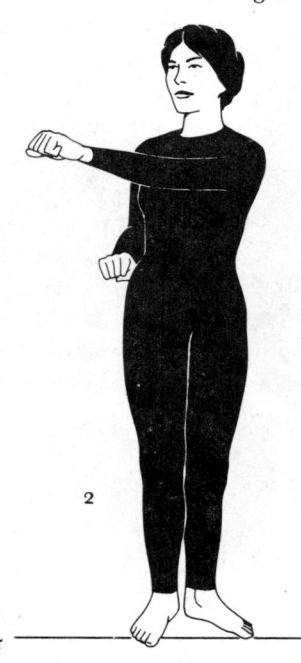

1

2

44

Yi Jin Jing — *Muscle Strengthening Exercises*

EXERCISE 10: *The hungry tiger jumping towards the food.*

This exercise strengthens the hands, arms and neck. It also develops flexibility of the hip and knee joints.

Caution: Those with hypertension are not permitted to do this exercise.

STARTING POSITION: Standing, feet together, arms at sides.

MOVEMENT: 1. Take a step forward with the right foot. Bend the right knee, while the left leg is stretched behind with the knee kept straight. Meanwhile, lean the body forward. Press the fingers to the ground. Raise the head a little, keeping the eyes wide open looking sternly straight ahead. 2. Slowly and slightly bend, then extend, both elbows simultaneously. When bending the elbows, the trunk falls and the head and chest move forward little, just like a tiger moving towards its food. When extending the elbows, the trunk rises again, and the head and chest move backward a little. Repeat 3–5 times, then stand up. Take a step back with the right foot, and return to the starting position.

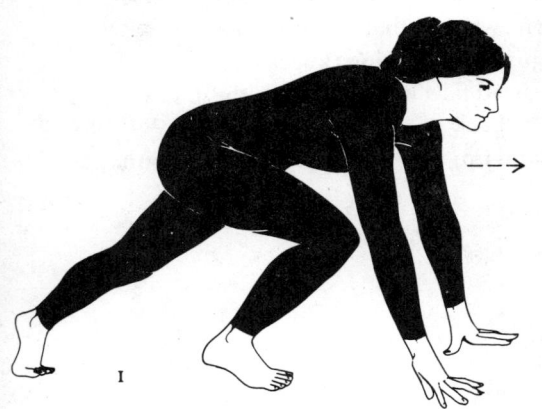

Repeat the above two movements, this time stepping forward with the left foot. This exercise is to be done only once.

Note: Breathe in as the head and chest move backward. As they move forward, breathe out.

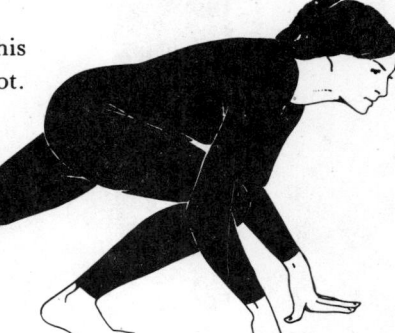

STARTING POSITION

TRADITIONAL CHINESE EXERCISES

EXERCISE II: *Bowing*.

This exercise develops flexibility of the spine and hip joints. It also helps prevent dizziness.

Caution: Avoid overstraining. Those with hypertension are not permitted to do this exercise.

STARTING POSITION: Standing, feet together, arms at sides.

MOVEMENT: 1. Place the hands at the back of the head, palms covering the ears. Extend the shoulders so that the elbows point outward. 2. Bend the trunk forward so that the head falls to the point in front of the knees, just as in bowing (knees kept straight). The degree to which the head falls will depend on the individual. In this position, tap the back of the head with the index fingers 10-20 times. Then stand up, slowly straightening the trunk, and return hands to sides.

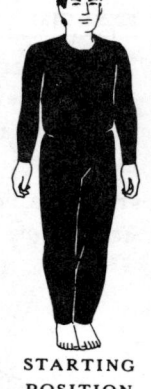

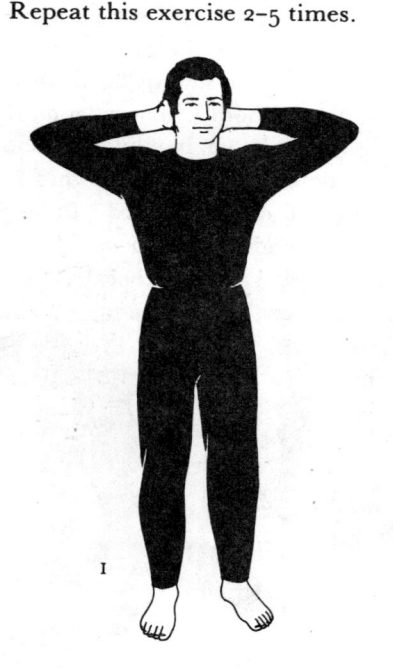

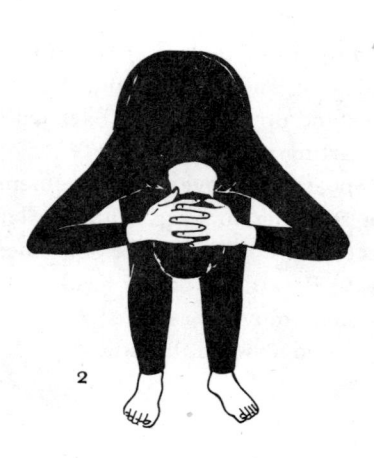

Repeat this exercise 2-5 times.

STARTING POSITION

Yi Jin Jing — *Muscle Strengthening Exercises*

EXERCISE 12: *Bending forward.*

This exercise develops flexibility of the spine and hip joints.

Caution: Avoid overstraining. Those with hypertension are not permitted to do this exercise.

STARTING POSITION: Standing, feet slightly apart, arms at sides.
MOVEMENT: 1. Raise the hands and push forward until the elbows are fully extended, palms forward. 2. Cross the hands, palms downward, while the arms are fully extended. Then bring the hands back in front of the chest. Uncross the hands. 3. The trunk bends forward and the hands push downward as much as possible. Raise the head, eyes straight ahead. Keep the knees straight. 4. Raise the trunk and stand up. Bend and extend the elbows seven times. 5. Finally, jump in place seven times with the arms hanging naturally.

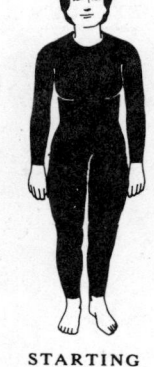

This completes the whole program of *Yi Jin Jing*.

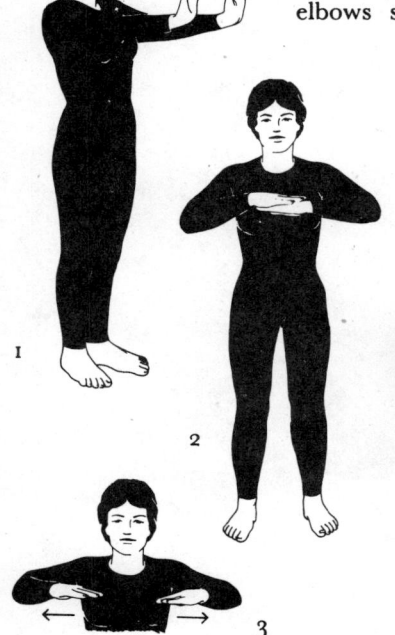

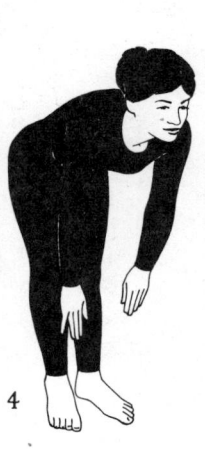

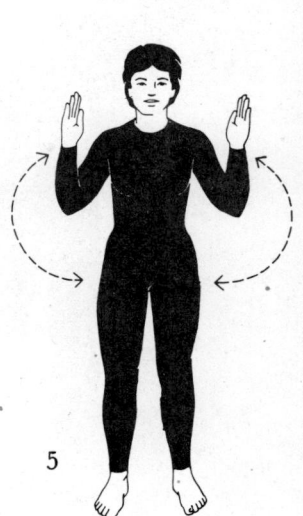

CHAPTER III

Ba Duan Jin — Eight Fine Exercises

Ba Duan Jin is a form of calisthenics which has been practiced in China for more than eight hundred years. It comprises eight exercises performed while standing. The traditional name of each exercise describes its movement and its effect on the body. Interestingly enough, the effects which are referred to coincide in part with modern concepts of exercise physiology.

Traditionally, *Ba Duan Jin* is performed with some effort or strain. However, the effort must be internal and not shown outwardly. Jerking movements and overstraining should be avoided. The advantage of *Ba Duan Jin* is that it is very effective in strengthening the arm and leg muscles, and in helping to develop the muscles of the chest, thus promoting good posture and helping to correct the defect of a rounded back. Because of this, it may be recommended for the youngster with weak muscles or defective posture. Modified *Ba Duan Jin* which is to be practiced gently without any effort or strain is suitable for the chronically ill and the elderly in poor physical condition. The traditional exercises of *Ba Duan Jin* are as follows:

TRADITIONAL CHINESE EXERCISES

EXERCISE 1: *Regulating the internal organs by raising both hands to the sky.*

This stretching exercise is good for improving posture. In addition, the movement of raising the arms is known to extend the range of vertical motion of the diaphragm, thus promoting deeper respiration, and providing soft "massage" to the stomach and intestines.

STARTING POSITION: Standing, heels together, arms at sides, eyes straight forward.

MOVEMENT: 1. Raise the arms from the sides slowly. Interlace the hands, and raise the heels about 2 inches (5 cm). 2. Turn the palms upward, and straighten out the elbows with effort. Raise the heels one inch higher. Hold this position for a while. 3. Unclasp the hands. Bring the arms down slowly. Keep heels raised. 4. Lower heels slowly. Repeat this exercise 8–16 times.

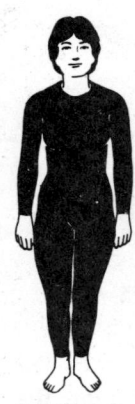

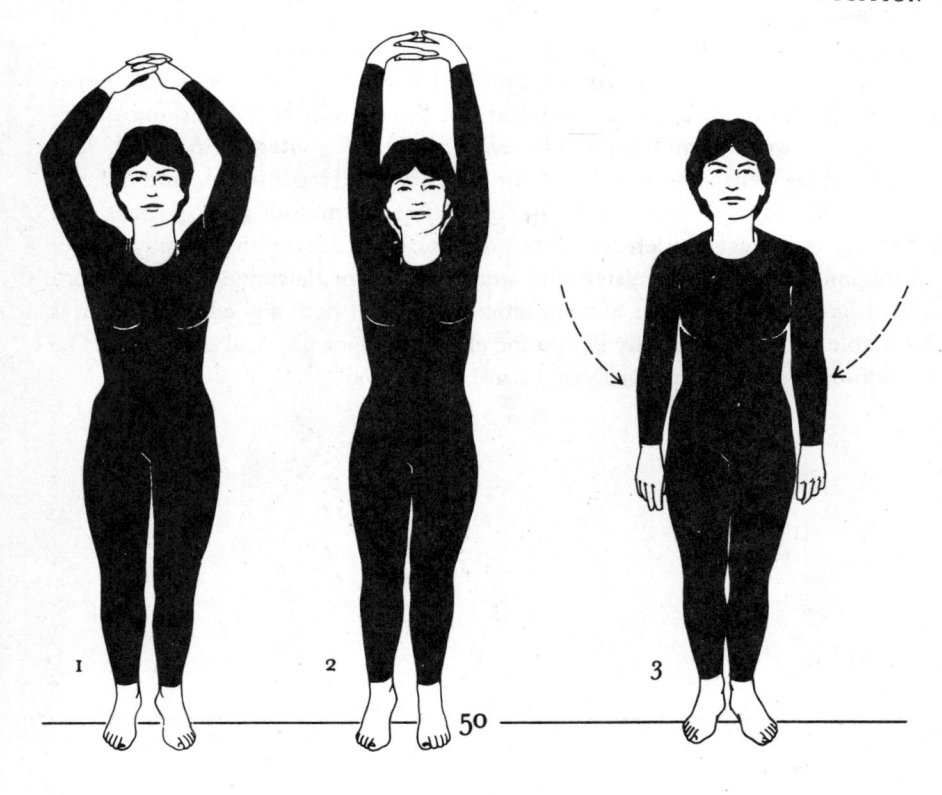

STARTING POSITION

Ba Duan Jin — *Eight Fine Exercises*

EXERCISE 2: *Shooting the eagle by drawing the bow with the hands.*

This exercise develops the muscles of the shoulder girdle and the sides of the chest. It is also good for strengthening the thighs.

STARTING POSITION: Standing, toes together.
MOVEMENT: 1. Take a step to the left with the left foot, keeping heels down, toes pointing forward. Bend the knees until the thighs are parallel to the ground, trunk erect. Cross the arms in front of the chest with the right arm outside the left, fingers spread. Turn the head to the left and look at the right hand. 2. Clench the left fist with the index finger pointing upward and the thumb pointing outward, palm facing left. Stretch the left arm slowly to the left until the elbow is fully extended. Meanwhile clench the right fist. Move the right arm slowly to

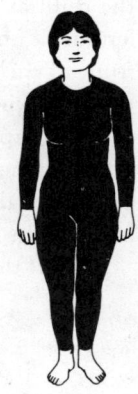

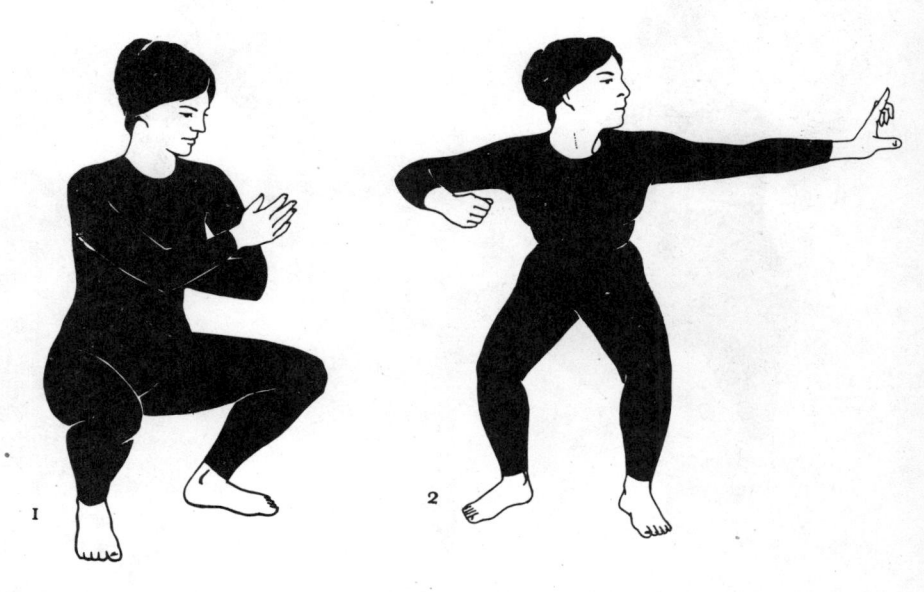

STARTING POSITION

1

2

the right as if drawing a bow; the right elbow pointing outward. Look at the left index finger. 3. Relax the arms and return them to the crossed position in front of the chest, with the left arm outside the right. Turn the head to the right, looking at the left hand. 4. Clench the right fist with the index finger pointing upward and the thumb pointing outward. Stretch the right arm slowly to the right until the elbow is fully extended. Meanwhile, clench the left fist. Move the left arm slowly to the left, and let the left elbow point outward. Look at the right index finger.

Repeat this exercise 8–16 times.

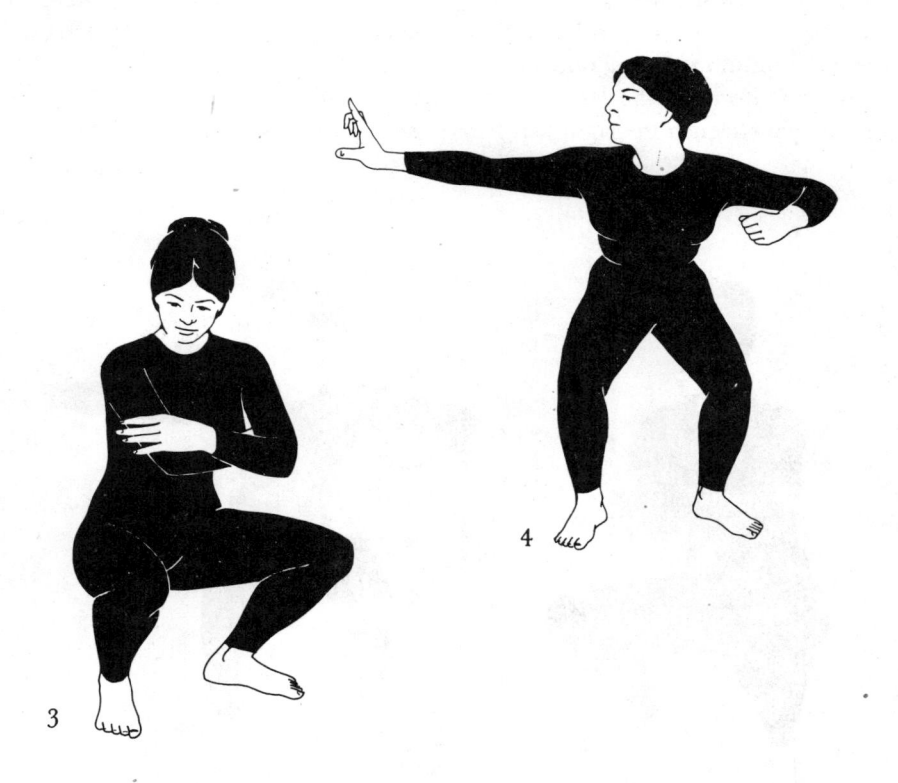

Ba Duan Jin — *Eight Fine Exercises*

EXERCISE 3: *Regulating the spleen and stomach by raising the hand upward.*

As in Exercise 1, this exercise increases the range of vertical motion of the diaphragm and helps regulate the digestion. It also develops the upper back, shoulders, and the back of the upper arms.

STARTING POSITION: Standing, arms at sides.
MOVEMENT: 1. Turn the left hand and raise it up from the side with the palm upward, fingers together and pointing to the right, elbow fully extended. Meanwhile, the right hand pushes downward with effort, palm down, fingers pointing forward. 2. Bring the left arm down to the starting position. The left hand pushes downward with effort, fingers pointing forward. Meanwhile, turn the right hand and raise it up from the side with the palm upward, fingers together and pointing to the left, elbow fully extended.

Repeat this exercise 8–16 times.

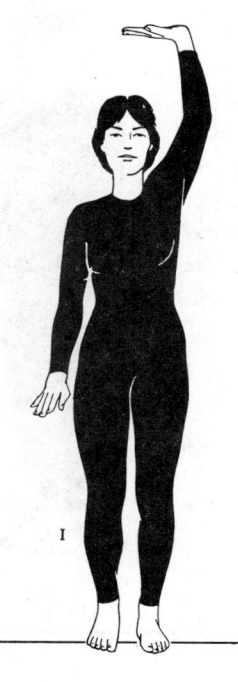

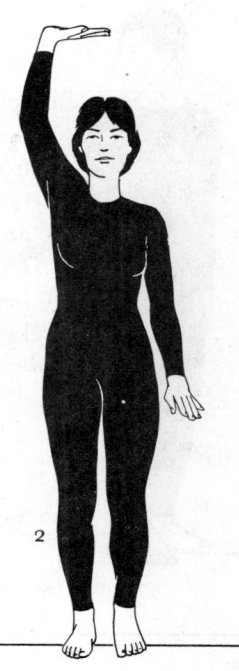

STARTING POSITION

EXERCISE 4: *Curing the five troubles and seven disorders* by turning the head backward and gazing sternly.*

This exercise is good for developing the neck. It is recommended for the prevention and treatment of neck pain or stiff neck due to rheumatism or degenerative disorders. It also helps relieve dizziness in patients with hypertension.

STARTING POSITION: Standing, head upright, arms at sides, palms pressing the thighs.

MOVEMENT: 1. Turn the head to the left slowly with the eyes looking sternly backward. Expand the chest with the shoulders slightly extended. Then return to the starting position, eyes straight ahead. 2. Turn the head to the right slowly with the eyes looking sternly backward. Expand the chest with the shoulders slightly extended. Again, return to the starting position, eyes straight ahead.

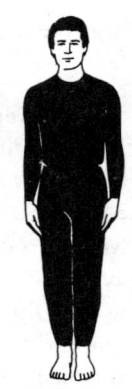

STARTING POSITION

Repeat this exercise 8–16 times.

*Note: The five troubles are troubles of the five organs: the heart, liver, spleen, lungs, and kidneys. The seven disorders are disorders arising from overeating, anger, overexertion, chilliness, extreme climate, anxiety, and apprehension. This exercise is said to cure these disorders because it promotes a sense of well-being.

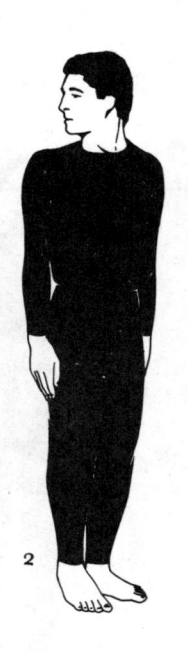

Ba Duan Jin — *Eight Fine Exercises*

EXERCISE 5: *Tranquilizing the fiery heart* by turning the head around and swinging the hips.*

This exercise strengthens the thighs and develops the flexibility of the spine.

STARTING POSITION: Stride standing (feet wide apart), knees bent, assume a horse-riding posture. Palms on the knees and thumbs pointing towards the body. Trunk erect.

MOVEMENT: 1. Bend the trunk and head low to the right, and then rotate the head in a small circle. Meanwhile, the hips swing slightly. Return to the starting position.

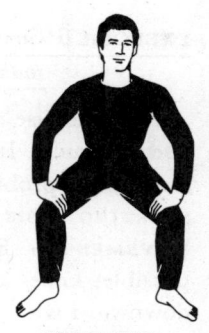

STARTING POSITION

2. Extend the trunk and the head to the left, and rotate the head in a small circle, then return to the starting position. Repeat the above two movements, rotating the head in the opposite direction.

Repeat the entire exercise 8–16 times.

**Note:* The term "fiery heart" refers to a group of symptoms arising from mental agitation, such as sleeplessness and restlessness. This exercise, like other moderate exercises, has the effect of regulating the psychological state, or "tranquilizing the fiery heart."

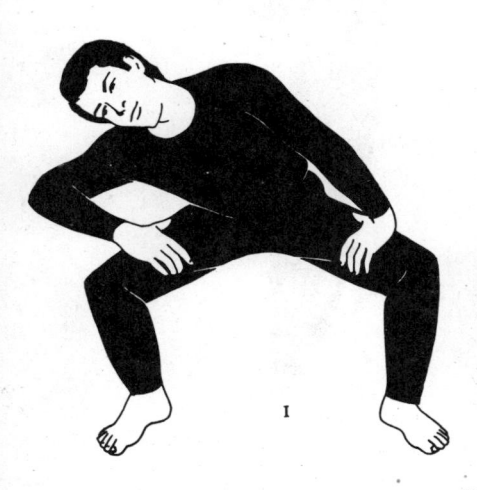

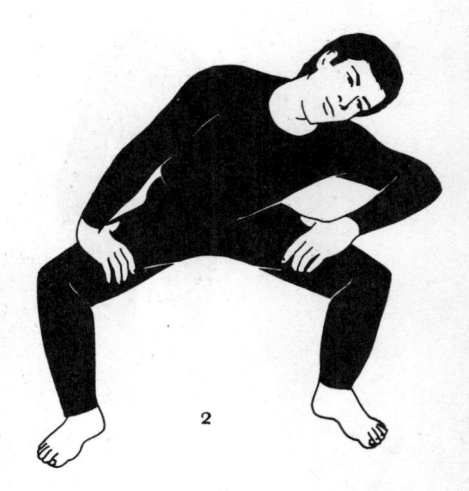

TRADITIONAL CHINESE EXERCISES

EXERCISE 6: *Strengthening the loins and kidneys by bending forward with hands touching the feet.*

This exercise develops the flexibility of the lumbar spine and hip joints. It helps in preventing backache. Those with lower back problems should not do this exercise.
STARTING POSITION: Standing.
MOVEMENT: 1. Bend the trunk forward slowly and as low as possible, knees kept straight. Meanwhile, stretch the arms downward with the hands touching or grasping the toes or ankles. Then raise the head slightly. Hold this position for a few seconds, then return to the starting position. 2. Extend the trunk backward with both hands placed on the lower back. Then return to the starting position.

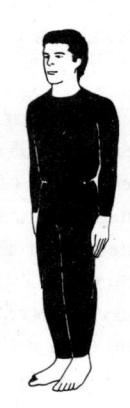

Repeat this exercise 8–16 times.

STARTING POSITION

1

2

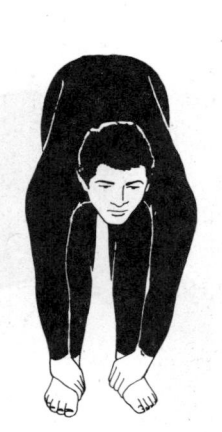

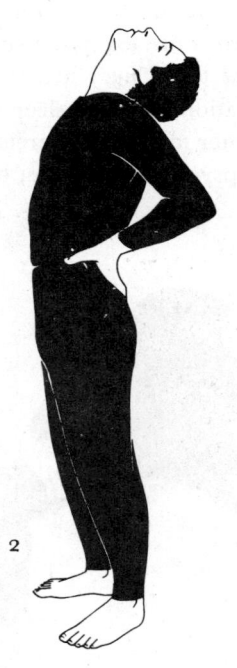

Ba Duan Jin — *Eight Fine Exercises*

EXERCISE 7: *Increasing the vital energy by tightening the fists and gazing sternly.*

This exercise develops the arms. Opening the eyes wide and gazing sternly are methods used traditionally to increase effort during the exercise.

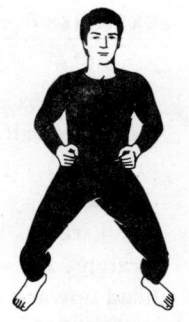

STARTING POSITION: Stride standing (feet separated shoulder width), knees bent, hands forming fists alongside the waist.

MOVEMENT: 1. Stretch the left arm forward as far as possible, fist tightened as if hitting a target, elbow fully extended. Meanwhile, clench the right fist with the elbow pointing backward. Eyes are kept wide open and gazing ahead sternly. 2. Bring the left fist back to the side of the waist, and stretch the right arm forward as far as possible, fist tightened as if hitting a target, elbow fully extended. Meanwhile, clench the left fist at the side of the waist with the elbow pointing backward. Eyes kept wide open and gazing ahead sternly. Then bring the right fist back to the side of the waist. Repeat this exercise 8–16 times.

EXERCISE 8: *Keeping all diseases away by raising the heels seven times.*

This exercise is good for improving posture and developing the calf muscles.

STARTING POSITION: Standing, toes together, palms on thighs.

MOVEMENT: 1. Expand the chest, keeping the knees straight. Raise the heels as high as possible and push the head upward with effort. 2. Lower the heels, returning to the starting position.

Repeat this exercise 8-16 times.

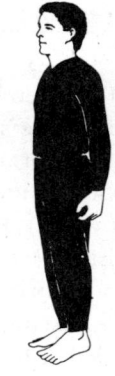

STARTING POSITION

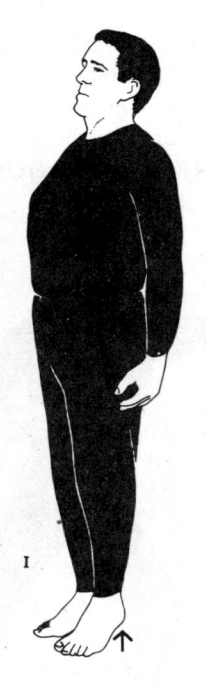

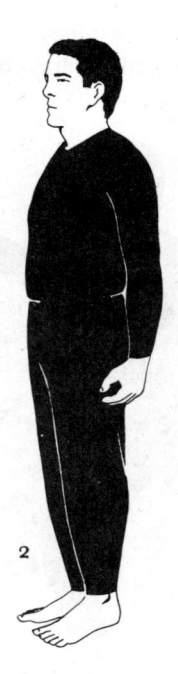

CHAPTER IV

Shier Duan Jin — Twelve Fine Exercises

Shier Duan Jin (Twelve Fine Exercises) is a traditional Chinese therapeutic exercise derived from the ancient *Tao Yin* (the Way of *Yin*). This program of exercise is a combination of bodily movements and self-administered massage. Usually the exercises are performed while sitting cross-legged on the floor or on a bed. Simple and effective, this program, through its invaluable therapeutic effects on the general well-being, is particularly suitable for the elderly and the chronically ill.

TRADITIONAL CHINESE EXERCISES

EXERCISE 1: *Biting the teeth.*

Close the mouth. Let the upper and lower teeth bite against each other. When doing this movement, open and close the jaw alternately. Repeat 20–30 times. It is said that this exercise prevents the teeth from becoming loose and is helpful in the treatment of periodontitis.

EXERCISE 2: *Moving the tongue around.*

Close the mouth. Move the tongue around, touching the gums and massaging the insides of the cheeks. This can stimulate the secretion of saliva and is said to have some therapeutic effect on gum inflammation and periodontitis.

EXERCISE 3: *"Washing" the face.*

Rub the hands together to warm the palms. Then "wash" the face by stroking it with the palms 20–30 times. It is said that this massage helps improve the circulation of blood to the skin, and maintain its elasticity and tone.

EXERCISE 4: *Beating the "drum of heaven."*

1. Put the hands on the back of the head, and cover your ears with the palms. Place the index fingers on the middle fingers. 2. Then slap the index fingers down to tap the back of the head (near the acupuncture point *feng chi*) 20–30 times. You may hear a sound of drumming. It is said that this massage may relieve headache and dizziness. According to traditional Chinese medicine, acupuncture on the *feng chi* point may cure headache and dizziness. Massage (percussion) on this point is expected to have a similar effect.

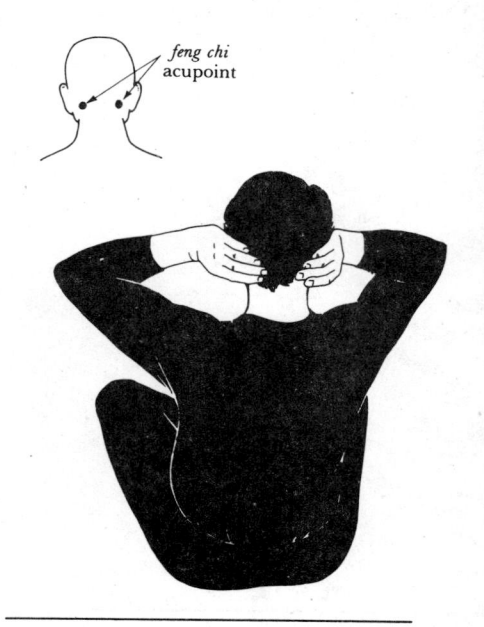

Shier Duan Jin — Twelve Fine Exercises

EXERCISE 5: *Winding the pulley.*

1. Starting with the elbows bent at a right angle beside the chest, and the forearms forward, clench the fists, palms downward. 2. Stretch the arms forward and upward, and then draw them downward and backward in a circular pattern, as in winding a wheel or a pulley. This circular movement of the shoulders is helpful for the prevention and treatment of periarthritis of the shoulder joints.

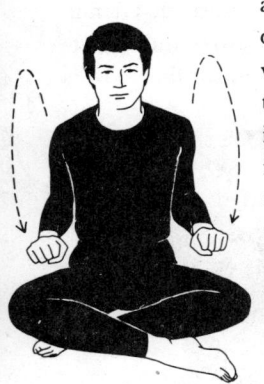

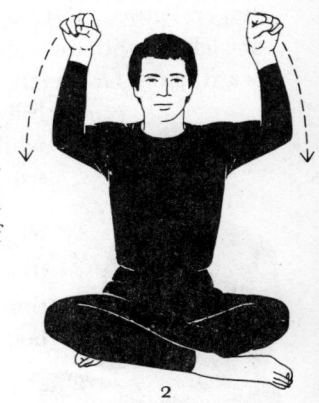

EXERCISE 6: *Pushing towards the sky.*

1. Interlace the hands in front of the abdomen, palms upward. 2. Raise the hands up above the head and turn the palms upward, making an effort to stretch the arms as if pushing towards the sky, elbows fully extended. Repeat 10–20 times. This is good for expanding the chest and strengthening the shoulder joints.

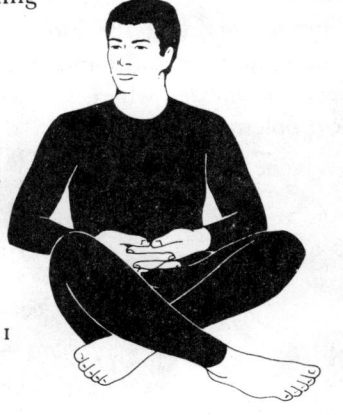

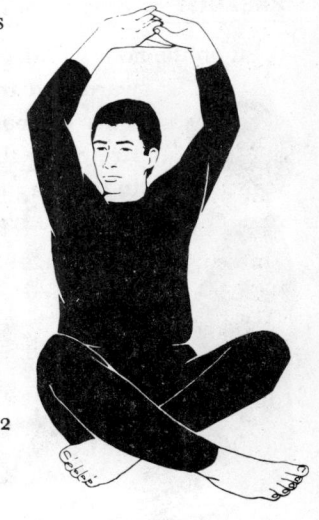

TRADITIONAL CHINESE EXERCISES

EXERCISE 7: *Drawing a bow.*

1. Cross the arms in front of the chest with the right arm outside the left, fingers spread. Turn the head to the left and look at the right hand. 2. Clench the left fist with the index finger pointing upward and the thumb pointing outward, palm facing left. Stretch the left arm slowly to the left until the elbow is fully extended. Meanwhile clench the right fist. Move the right arm slowly to the right as in drawing a bow. Repeat this movement 10–20 times. The effects on the body are similar to those of Exercise 6.

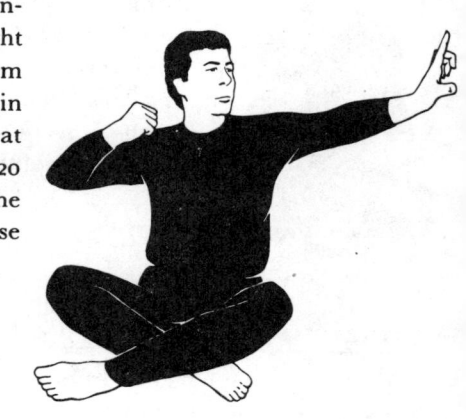

EXERCISE 8: *Bending the trunk with the hands touching the feet.*

1. Sit on the floor with legs kept straight (long sitting). 2. Bend the trunk forward and touch the feet with the hands. Repeat 10–20 times. This is good for maintaining the mobility of the spine and stretching the back muscles and hamstrings. However, sitting in this way is contraindicated where there is a back problem.

Shier Duan Jin — *Twelve Fine Exercises*

EXERCISE 9: *Stroking the* dan tian* *(field of pills).*

Dan tian is a traditional acupoint located about 2 inches below the umbilicus. In practice, stroking the *dan tian* is almost the same as stroking the lower abdomen. The massage is performed with three fingers of the right hand. Acupuncture on this point is indicated in cases of indigestion, lower abdominal pain, and excessive nocturnal emissions, and massage over this point is expected, and has been observed, to relieve the aforementioned symptoms. Massage for five minutes.

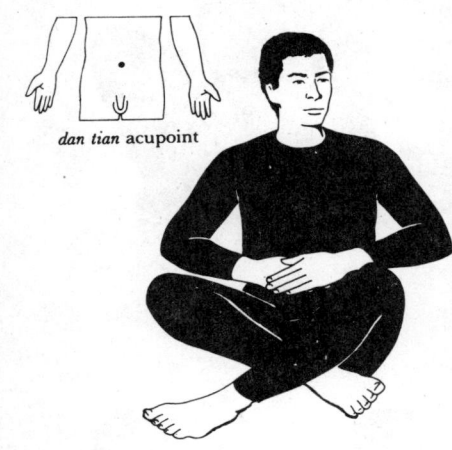

dan tian acupoint

**Note:* In Chinese, the word *dan* means pill, and *tian* means field. The ancient Chinese scholars noted that when one meditates, focusing the awareness on the center of the lower abdomen, one can sense a "warm pool" forming in that area. This small pool of warmth is said to be a valuable "pill." And so *dan tian* is called the "field of pills."

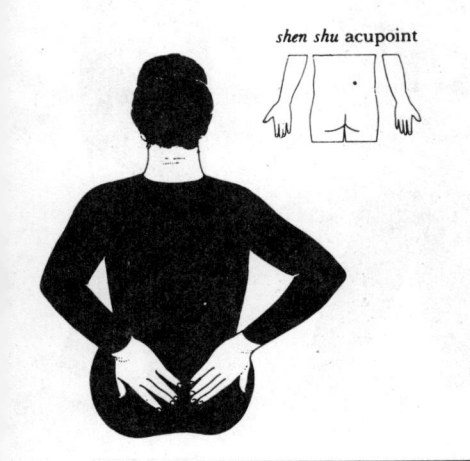

shen shu acupoint

EXERCISE 10: *Stroking the* shen shu *(kidney point).*

Rub the hands together to warm the palms. Then stroke the lower back with both hands for five minutes. The point *shen shu* is located on the lower back. Acupuncture or massage on this point has a preventive and therapeutic effect for backache caused by straining the back muscles.

TRADITIONAL CHINESE EXERCISES

EXERCISE 11: *Stroking the yung chuan.*

Rub the hands together to warm the fingers. Then stroke the left sole with three fingers of the right hand until there is a feeling of warmth in the sole. Then, stroke the right sole with the left hand. The acupoint *yung chuan* is on the sole of the foot. Massage on this point is helpful in the treatment of insomnia and palpitation, and is good for strengthening the feet as well.

yung chuan acupoint

EXERCISE 12: *Stretching the legs.*

Stand. Taking a step backward, stretch the left leg. Then return to the starting position. Do the same with the right leg. Repeat this exercise 10–20 times. This exercise improves the blood circulation in the legs and helps relax the muscles.

The above exercises and massage may be practiced in the morning after getting up and/or in the evening before going to sleep. They may be practiced in the complete series or selectively, that is, only some of them per session. One may establish one's own priority according to symptoms, as well as vary the number of repetitions or time allotted each exercise in a given routine.

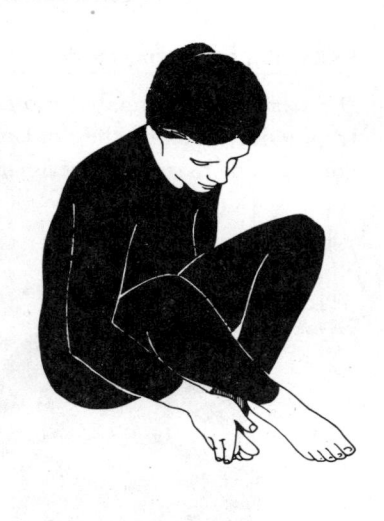

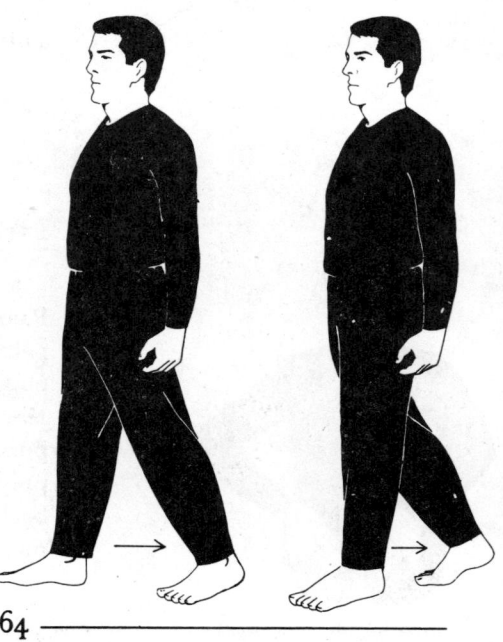

CHAPTER V

Chi Kung—Invigorating Exercises

Chi Kung is a special form of traditional Chinese exercise. The Chinese term *Chi* means the air one breathes in and out. It also refers to the vitality or energy in the body. The term *Kung* means exercise, skill, or training. Translated literally, then, *Chi Kung* is a breath-training or invigorating exercise. Essentially, *Chi Kung* is an exercise which combines breathing with meditation and relaxation.

Technically, the practice of *Chi Kung* has three aspects: adjusting the posture, adjusting the breathing, and adjusting the mind. These three elements are closely associated with each other, and mastering *Chi Kung* means learning and mastering the techniques of these "three adjustments."

In China, *Chi Kung* is used widely to treat a number of diseases and to promote longevity. Scientific studies have shown that *Chi Kung* is quite effective in preserving the energy of the body. It may be called an "energy-saving" exercise. *Chi Kung* is also renowned for its remarkable capacity for bringing relaxation to both mind and body. It is thus a good remedy for many of the stress-related diseases. In addition, through the mechanical action of the *Chi Kung* breathing exercises, the internal organs benefit greatly since the exercises provide an "internal massage."

In China, many kinds of *Chi Kung* are practiced. Today the most popular forms are *Chi Kung for Relaxation*, *Chi Kung for Fitness*, and *Chi Kung for the Internal Organs*. The methods and applications of these three are described in this section.

TRADITIONAL CHINESE EXERCISES

How to practice *Chi Kung* correctly

In order to benefit from *Chi Kung* the following principles must be observed.
- *Relaxation, quiet, and ease:* During the practice, relax both body and mind. First of all, loosen the belt and clothing. Relax the body; drop the shoulders, keeping the chest in. This posture is maintained without any effort. If uncomfortable, continue to readjust the posture until the muscles of the entire body, especially those of the abdomen, are relaxed. Then relax the mind, letting it dwell on pleasant and peaceful things. All anxiety and unhappiness should be kept out. Focus attention on the practice, and then adjust your breathing. Smooth and easy breathing will help the body to relax better. A sense of relaxation during exhalation may be experienced.

  Quietness and stillness require concentration of the mind. Attention is focused on the practice of *Chi Kung* without other thoughts interfering. When entering the state of quietness and stillness, one will feel a sense of emptiness in the mind. Sensations resulting from external stimulation (sound, light) become weaker. Sometimes the limbs seem to no longer exist or to not be where they are.

  At the initial stage, a beginner may find it hard to concentrate. Irrelevant and random thoughts emerge now and then, and make him or her vexed and uneasy. If this happens, relax and quiet yourself with auto-suggestion such as "My thoughts are turned inward and I am at ease." After a period of training, you will gradually succeed in calming down and entering a state of inward quietness, feeling serene and still.
- *Integrating breath with concentration:* During the practice of *Chi Kung*, the training of concentration and regulation of respiration should be combined. Breathing is directed by thought which controls its rhythm, depth, and speed, constantly directing it in and out.

  The essence of training one's concentration consists of turning towards an inward quietness. Regulation of the breathing aims at developing a pattern of smooth, deep, slow, and rhythmic breathing, done easily and without hoarseness. Breath-training is especially emphasized in *Chi Kung*

Chi Kung — *Invigorating Exercises*

for the Internal Organs, while *Chi Kung for Fitness* and *Chi Kung for Relaxation* emphasize the training of concentration.

- *Alternating stillness with activity:* *Chi Kung* is a form of physical training requiring little motion of the body, so it is advisable, if possible, to also participate in other therapeutic exercises and sports. Generally, active exercises are scheduled to follow *Chi Kung*.
- *Gradual progress:* *Chi Kung* is an art and skill. A long time is required to master its special method. Only patience and gradual progression will lead to success. The introduction to quietness and the training of breath should begin with simple methods and then gradually proceed to more demanding and complex methods. The length of a *Chi Kung* session usually begins with fifteen to twenty minutes, gradually increasing to between thirty and forty-five minutes.

Apart from the aformentioned principles, there are some maxims which a *Chi Kung* participant should follow:

Stop all reading and recreational activities between ten and fifteen minutes before a session, so as to bring the body and mind to a quieter state. This is important if one is to experience a successful *Chi Kung* session.

The duration of each session is best determined by the participant. When it is felt that the session should come to an end, open the eyes slowly, rub the face with the hands, and then stand up and do some stretching exercises.

Because it would be difficult to concentrate, *Chi Kung* should not be practiced when feeling hungry, nor after a full meal. The same is true in cases of fever, bad colds, diarrhea, and the like.

The possible side effects of *Chi Kung*

It is quite safe to practice *Chi Kung for Relaxation, Chi Kung for Fitness,* and *Chi Kung for the Internal Organs,* because if practiced correctly, these three kinds of *Chi Kung* will not cause any undue side effects. Beginners, however, may find it difficult to get used to the particular position, breathing, and concentration demanded by *Chi Kung*. In addition, lack of proficiency in the skill of

Chi Kung will sometimes cause abnormal responses in the body during the performance. Unfavorable reactions such as the following may be prevented or overcome by taking suitable measures.

- Backache after prolonged sitting. This is the result of malposition in sitting. For those who have had back problems, it is advisable to begin the practice in a lying position, and gradually shift to a sitting one. The length of each session may be cut down by those who feel discomfort in the back.
- Numbness of the legs when sitting cross-legged. This may be prevented by bending and stretching the legs immediately before assuming the cross-legged sitting position. If numbness occurs in the course of sitting, it is advisable to massage the legs or adjust the position to make the legs feel at ease, or to stand up and stretch the legs. If the numbness disappears, the participant may return to the original sitting position.
- Discomfort and shortness of breath. This may be seen in beginners, when they try to do very deep breathing. Malposition and poor motivation also may produce discomfort and difficulty in concentrating. Appropriate adjustment of respiration and position will help produce a state of calm and make breathing easier.
- A suffocating feeling in the chest, and pain over the lower costal (rib) region. This may be caused by inappropriate respiration — holding the breath in the throat or chest. If this occurs, the participant should change the breathing pattern by not holding the breath.
- Drowsiness and even falling asleep. This may come about when in a lying position. If so, a sitting position should be taken instead, with the eyes open, focused gently on the tip of the nose. A cup of hot tea or a short walk around the room will also help one keep alert.
- Strange sensations. Sometimes, during profound *Chi Kung* relaxation, one may experience a sensation of numbness, scorching, itching, or a flow of warmth in the skin or in the muscles of certain parts of the body. There is no cause for alarm when this occurs. The strange sensation will disappear or be reduced if one focuses attention on the lower abdomen.
- Palpitation. This may arise from hyperventilation or prolonged breath

Chi Kung — *Invigorating Exercises*

holding, or emotional tension. If one strives to find the cause one can then remove it.
- Headache and fainting. These may be caused by strained breathing or emotional upset. Again, it is necessary to find the cause in order to remove it.
- Discomfort in the head due to pulsation of the temporal artery. This occurs sometimes when practicing *Chi Kung* while lying on one's side. The discomfort will be removed by adjusting the position of the head so that the temporal region is not pressed firmly.

Chi Kung for Relaxation: Method and Application

Chi Kung for Relaxation is relatively simple to perform. It is indicated for chronic diseases in general.

POSITION: Lying on the back, with high pillows under the head. The shoulders and upper back are supported by towels or soft pads. The head is kept straight in line with the body. Arms are at the sides and relaxed. Legs are kept straight. Eyes, slightly closed. The mouth is shut with the upper and lower teeth touching, and the tip of the tongue placed against the roof of the mouth.

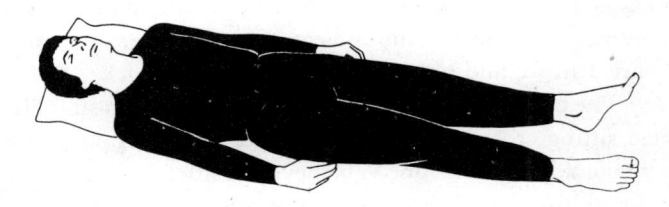

RESPIRATION: Breathe naturally through the nose. Regulate the breathing and let it be fine (not hoarse), rhythmic in speed and depth, and steady (without jerking or blocking).

RELAXATION: Use a cue word to induce the relaxation response. The participant is to mentally repeat, first the word "quiet" with each inhalation, then the word "relaxed" with each exhalation. Thinking about the word "relaxed," deliberately relax a part of the body at the same time. Thus, for each breath a part of the body is to be relaxed. The procedure begins with the head. After the head is relaxed, relax in turn, the arms, hands, chest, abdomen, upper back, lower back, hips and buttocks, legs, and finally the feet. After that, scan over the whole body to see whether there are any specific regions which may still be tense. If there are, make some adjustment to allow that region to be relaxed. After all muscles are relaxed, focus on the blood vessels, then the nerves, and finally, the internal organs (especially the affected organs), imagining each of these being relaxed. Such a use of imagery has been found to bring about a sense of relaxation in the areas where the attention is focused.

FREQUENCY AND LENGTH OF TRAINING: These depend on the individual. Generally speaking, hospitalized patients are required to practice three or four 30-minute sessions daily. Others who do not have sufficient time to do this are advised to practice one or two 30-minute sessions daily. The course of *Chi Kung* therapy varies. Generally, it takes 3-4 months to obtain significant therapeutic results.

Chi Kung for Fitness: Method and Application

Chi Kung for Fitness emphasizes the training of concentration to attain an inward quietness. It is principally indicated for hypertension, the psychoneuroses, heart disease, and pulmonary emphysema.

POSITION: The position commonly adopted is sitting on a stool. It may also be performed sitting cross-legged or standing. Patients in poor physical condition may take a lying position. Whichever position is chosen, keep the eyes slightly closed, the mouth shut with the upper and lower teeth touching, and the tip of the tongue placed against the hard palate.

Chi Kung — *Invigorating Exercises*

1. *Sitting on a stool.* Sit on a big stool, feet apart and touching the floor. The knees are bent at a right angle. The trunk remains straight. The thighs are parallel to the floor with the hips bent at a right angle. The palms are placed on the thighs comfortably, with the elbows bent slightly. The head is kept straight. Drop the shoulders and hold in the chest.

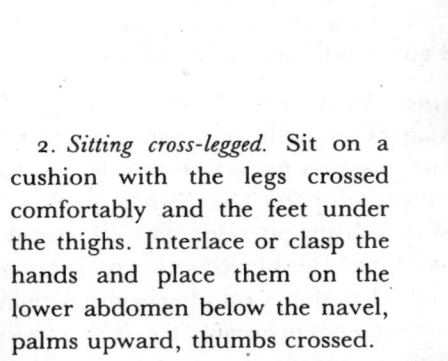

2. *Sitting cross-legged.* Sit on a cushion with the legs crossed comfortably and the feet under the thighs. Interlace or clasp the hands and place them on the lower abdomen below the navel, palms upward, thumbs crossed.

3. *Standing.* Since the position of standing consumes more energy and requires more effort, it is indicated only for patients in moderately good condition. Stand on the floor, feet apart, toes pointing forward and slightly inward, knees slightly bent. Keep the trunk straight. Raise the arms to shoulder level. Bend and drop the elbow slightly as if the arms are circling a big tree. Flex the fingers slightly as if holding a ball in the hand.

TRADITIONAL CHINESE EXERCISES

RESPIRATION: Use either diaphragmatic breathing or chest-abdominal breathing.

1. *Diaphragmatic breathing.* When breathing in, expand and protrude the abdomen; when breathing out, contract the abdomen, pressing it down. The breathing gradually becomes deeper and deeper until a rate of six to eight breaths per minute is attained. Breathe comfortably and easily, without any strain.

2. *Chest-abdominal breathing.* As in *Chi Kung for Relaxation,* breathe naturally through the nose. Regulate the breathing and let it be fine (not hoarse), rhythmic in speed and depth, and steady (without jerking or blocking).

QUIETNESS TRAINING: To induce the state of inward quietness, the basic method is to focus attention on the lower abdomen. As a preparatory or introductory procedure, one may begin by counting breaths, then following the breath with one's attention. After two or three weeks of training, one may change the method to focusing attention on the lower abdomen.

Counting the breaths. One begins by counting one's breaths. Each breath includes inhalation and exhalation. Counting begins with number one (the first breath counted), and proceeds to number ten. The counting is repeated again from one to ten, until one can concentrate fully, and gradually enters a state of inward quietness. If the counting is interrupted by irrelevant drifting thoughts, one should draw one's attention back and focus it on counting again from the very beginning.

Following the breath. Let your attention follow the descent of the inhaled air from the nose down into the lung, and then the ascent of the exhaled air from the lung up to the nose. This method is more natural than counting breaths. Yet it may still be interrupted and one's thoughts may be attracted outward, drifting far off. If this occurs, one should draw the attention inward again and focus it on the movement of the inhaled and exhaled air.

Focusing the attention on the lower abdomen. Thought is lightly and gently focused on the lower abdomen about two inches below the navel. The "attachment" of one's thought should be loose and done without any reluctance or stress. If this "attachment" is broken by the interference of drifting thoughts, draw the attention inward and again "attach" it to the lower abdomen.

FREQUENCY AND LENGTH OF TRAINING: As in *Chi Kung for Relaxation,* these depend on the individual. Generally speaking, hospitalized patients are required to practice for 30 minutes, 3-4 times daily. Others who do not have time for 3 or 4 sessions, should practice once or twice daily, for 30 minutes each.

The following table outlines the program used in teaching patients in the *Chi Kung for Fitness* class at Zhong Shan Medical College Hospital.

Table 1. Program for the Practice of *Chi Kung for Fitness*

Stage	First Stage (1st week)	Second Stage (2nd-4th week)	Third Stage (5th week)
Position:	Lying or sitting.	Sitting on stool or sitting cross-legged.	Sitting or standing.
Respiration:	Natural, deep breathing.	Diaphragmatic breathing (deep).	Diaphragmatic breathing (deep).
Inducing quietness:	Counting breaths and following the breath.	Following the breath. Focusing attention on the lower abdomen.	Focusing attention on the lower abdomen.
Frequency and length:	3-4 sessions/day, 15-20 mins. per session.	3-4 sessions/day, 30 mins. per session.	3-4 sessions/day, 30-45 mins. per session.
Requirements:	1. Correct posture. 2. Smooth, rhythmic, and steady breathing. 3. Focusing attention on the breath.	1. Correct posture. 2. Smooth, rhythmic, deep, and steady breathing. 3. Inward quietness.	1. Correct posture. 2. Smooth, deep, rhythmic, slow, steady, and relaxed breathing. 3. Profound inward quietness. 4. Relief of symptoms. 5. Interest in *Chi Kung*.

TRADITIONAL CHINESE EXERCISES

Chi Kung for the Internal Organs: Method and Application

The method of *Chi Kung for the Internal Organs* emphasizes training of the breath. It is indicated in the treatment of peptic ulcer, viral hepatitis, chronic constipation, and gastroptosis (downward displacement of the stomach).

POSITION: Preferably lying on the side or sitting on a stool.

1. *Lying on the side.* In general, lying on the right side is preferable, with the head slightly bent forward, the right hand placed on a pillow about three inches from the head, palm upward. The left arm is extended comfortably with the hand placed on the left hip, palm downward. Both legs are bent comfortably. The left leg is placed on the right leg. The mouth is shut with the upper and lower teeth touching, the tip of the tongue placed against the hard palate. Keep the eyes slightly closed.

Note: Those who feel a pulsation of the artery on the side of the head, while practicing *Chi Kung* in this position, may instead adopt the position of lying on the back: Lying on the back, with high pillows under the head, keep the shoulders and upper back supported by towels or soft pads. The head is kept straight in line with the body. Arms are at the sides and relaxed. Legs are kept straight. The eyes, mouth, and tongue are the same as above.

2. *Sitting on a stool.* Sit on a big stool, feet apart and touching the floor. The knees are bent at a right angle. The trunk remains straight. The thighs are parallel to the floor with the hips bent at a right angle. The palms are placed on the thighs comfortably with the elbows bent slightly. The head is kept straight, with the shoulders dropped and the chest held in. The eyes, mouth, and tongue are the same as in Position 1, above.

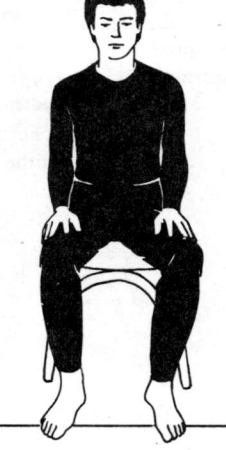

Chi Kung — *Invigorating Exercises*

RESPIRATION: Utilizing the pattern of interval respiration, the patient is asked to pause and hold between each breath. The breathing is diaphragmatic and through the nose. The pattern of breathing is as follows:

Inhale – exhale – pause. Hold the breath, raise the tongue, and concentrate on some words in the mind. Lower the tongue – inhale...and so on.

While holding the breath, interrupt the respiratory movement for a while and focus the attention on the lower abdomen. Never strenuously, close off the air at the throat or at the upper abdomen. With continued practice the time of the interval between each breath will gradually lengthen. This may be helped by reciting a phrase silently, usually one word per second. In general, it is advisable to recite 3–7 words during each interval, since the length of holding the breath will be 3–7 seconds. The content of the phrase should be self-chosen and should have a positive impact. For example, at the initial stage, one may recite "Quietness is fine," that is, three words for holding the breath for three seconds. Later, "Quietness and relaxation are wonderful" (five words, when holding the breath for five seconds), and then, "Quietness and relaxation give me perfect health" (seven words, when holding the breath for seven seconds). The psychological effects of interrupted respiration are not yet clearly understood. It is possible that interrupted breathing induces regular changes in abdominal pressure, which then can stimulate the blood circulation in the abdominal cavity and improve the movement of the bowels.

QUIETNESS TRAINING: By reciting phrases mentally, in order to focus attention on the breath, one becomes relaxed in both mind and body, enabling one to expel any irrelevant thoughts and to gradually enter a state of inward quietness.

CHAPTER VI

Other Traditional Chinese Exercises

TRADITIONAL CHINESE EXERCISES

Breathing exercise

This dynamic breathing exercise is done with large-ranging movements of the limbs and trunk. As a type of calisthenics, it has been observed to have a beneficial effect on general physical well-being, and to be helpful in the treatment of some chronic diseases, such as hypertension.

STARTING POSITION: Standing, relaxed, feet apart, arms at sides.

MOVEMENT: 1. Raise the arms forward and upward slowly until they reach a vertical position, with fingers extended. Breathe in. 2. Squat with the knees bent and bring the arms slowly down to the sides, and breathe out. Return to the position in step 1, breathing in. Then squat again, breathing out.

Repeat this exercise 10–20 times.

For the advanced practitioner, the exercise of twisting the body may be added to the above movements. (See Exercise 22, page 152.)

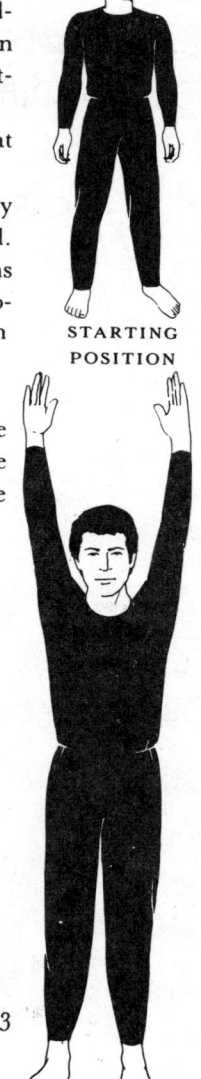

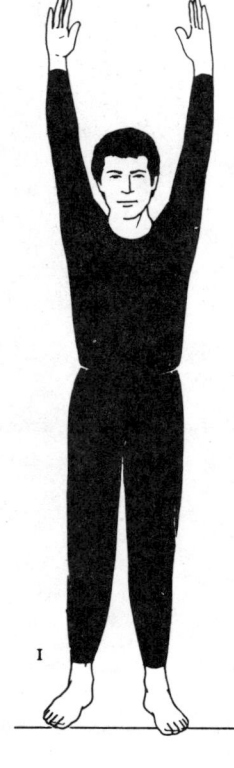

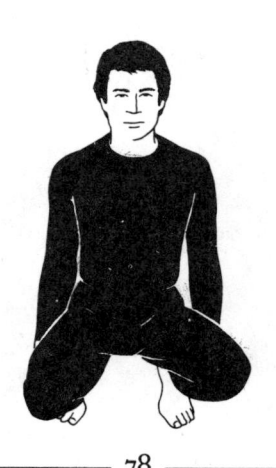

STARTING POSITION

Other Traditional Chinese Exercises

Exercise with the *Tai Chi* Stick

The *Tai Chi* Stick exercise is one of China's most ancient calisthenics. Like *Tai Chi Chuan*, it is gentle in nature, demanding that the participant be relaxed, quiet, and composed throughout the exercise. It may be used in the treatment of the psychoneuroses, peptic ulcer, and other chronic diseases.

EXERCISE 1: *Circling at a resting position.*

STARTING POSITION: Standing (feet apart), sitting on a stool, or lying on one's back. Elbows bent, fingers slightly flexed, palms holding a stick about 14 inches (35 cm) long at both ends, body relaxed, eyes partly closed. Focus attention on the lower abdomen. Breathe in and out smoothly.

MOVEMENT: With the stick held between the two palms, draw a circle in front of the abdomen, like a wheel rolling incessantly, at the rate of 40–50 cycles per minute.

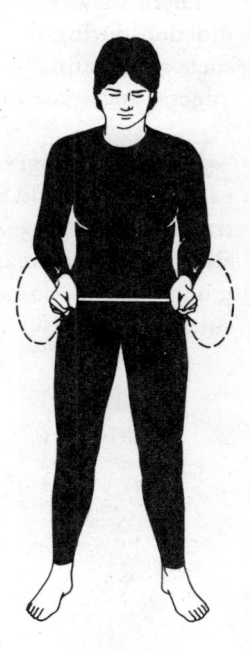

EXERCISE 2: *Circling while moving the legs up and down.*

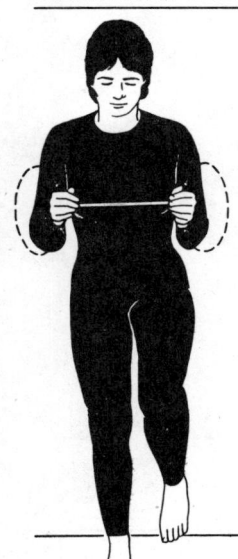

STARTING POSITION: Standing.
MOVEMENT: Bend the left leg upward and, at the same time, draw a circle with the stick held between the two palms. Lower the left foot and draw a circle with the stick. Bend the right leg upward and, at the same time, draw a circle. Lower the right foot and, at the same time, draw a circle.

EXERCISE 3: *Circling while walking.*

STARTING POSITION: Standing.
MOVEMENT: Step forward, and circle with both hands at the same time, the stick held between the palms. The rate is one circle for each step.

There may be various responses of the bodily function during the practice of the *Tai Chi* Stick, such as sweating, a sensation of warmth on the fingers, and sometimes twitching of the muscles.

Precaution: Progress gradually. For a beginner, each session should last about 2–5 minutes. After a training period of 3–4 weeks, the length of each session may be increased to 5–10 minutes. After a month or two, 10–20 minutes for each session is suitable.

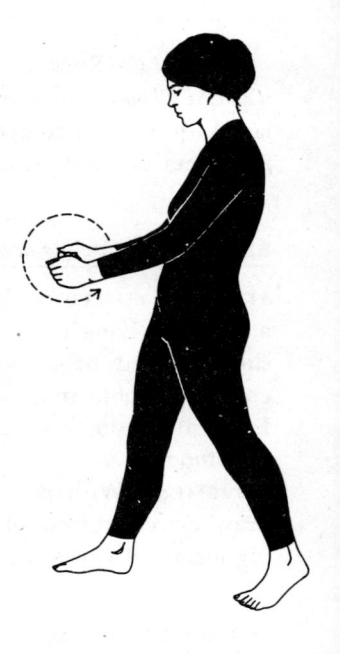

PART II
Chinese Fitness Exercises

CHAPTER VII

Fitness Exercises for Children

This program is good for children (age 7-15), to develop cardiorespiratory fitness, flexibility, and good posture.

CHINESE FITNESS EXERCISES

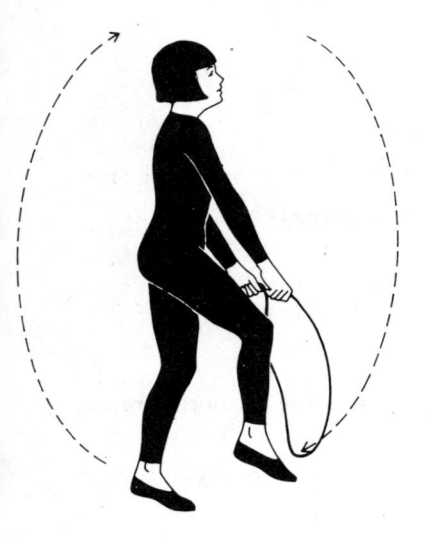

EXERCISE 1: *Rope jumping.*

PURPOSE: To develop the heart and lungs.
STARTING POSITION: Standing with a rope held in the hands.
MOVEMENT: 1. Free skipping with a rope 25–50 times. 2. Skipping the rope on the spot 25–50 times with jogging steps. 3. Skipping the rope on the spot 25–50 times, feet together.

Rest one minute between each of the above.

This sequence may be repeated three times.

EXERCISE 2: *Hitting the bean bag.*

PURPOSE: To develop strength in the upper arms.
STARTING POSITION: Standing before a bean bag, fists clenched.
MOVEMENT: Stretch out the arms and punch the bean bag with the left and right fists alternately.

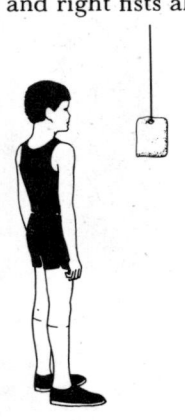

STARTING POSITION

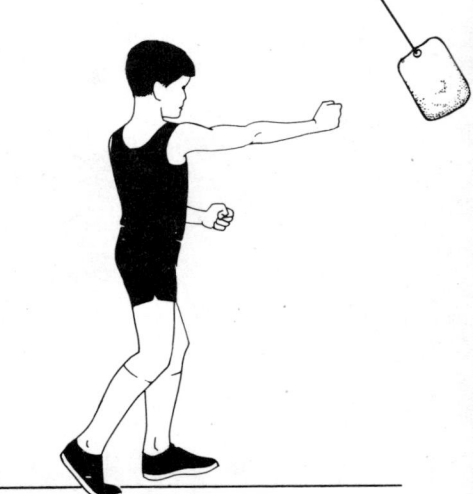

Fitness Exercises for Children

EXERCISE 3: *Monkey play.*

PURPOSE: To develop agility.
STARTING POSITION: Standing, feet apart, arms hanging naturally at the sides.
MOVEMENT: 1. Jump forward with the left foot landing on the ground, while the right foot remains suspended in the air with the knee slightly bent. At the same time, reach forward with the left hand, fingers firmly held together, to imitate the picking movement of a monkey. The right arm is slightly bent at the side. Then jump backward and return to the starting position. 2. Jump forward with the right foot landing on the ground, while the left foot remains suspended with the knee slightly bent. At the same time, reach forward with the right hand, fingers firmly held together, to imitate the picking movement of a monkey. The left arm is slightly bent at the side. Then jump backward and return to the starting position.

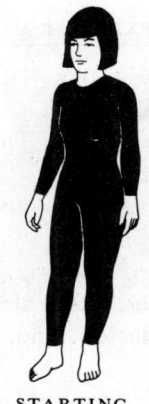

Repeat this exercise 8–10 times.

Note: This exercise should be performed in a swift and lively manner, just as a monkey might do it.

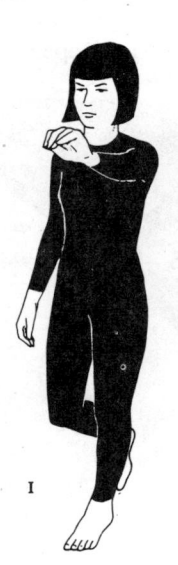

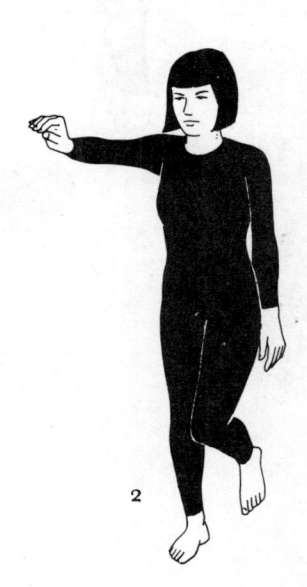

CHINESE FITNESS EXERCISES

EXERCISE 4: *Tiger walking.*

PURPOSE: To develop the flexibility of the lumbar spine and hip joints.

Caution: This exercise is not suitable for children with back injuries.

STARTING POSITION: Standing with feet separated shoulder width.

MOVEMENT: 1. Bend the trunk forward, bending the knees so the back is almost parallel to the floor. Grasp the left ankle with the left hand, and the right ankle with the right hand. 2. Take a step forward with the right foot, while turning the head to the right. 3. Then take a step forward with the left foot, while turning the head to the left. Walk 8 steps in this manner. Then raise the trunk and return to the starting position. Breathe naturally in a rhythmic manner 8-10 times.

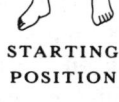

Repeat this exercise 2-4 times.

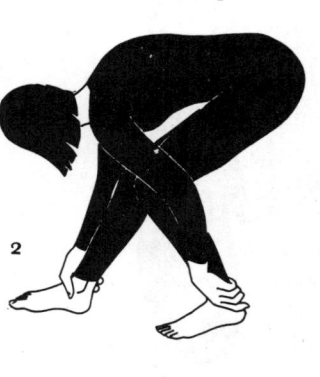

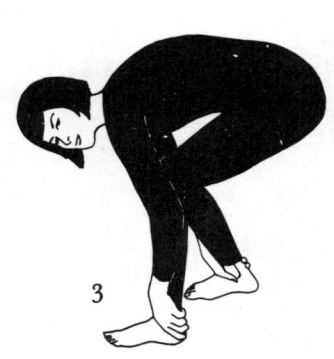

STARTING POSITION

EXERCISE 5: *Worm wriggling*.

PURPOSE: To develop the muscles of the back and to prevent scoliosis.
STARTING POSITION: Lying on the back, arms at sides, feet together.
MOVEMENT: Move the body along the floor in the direction of the head by shrugging the shoulders for 2-3 minutes.

Note: The movement of the body looks like the wriggling of a worm. Do not use the hands to assist the movement.

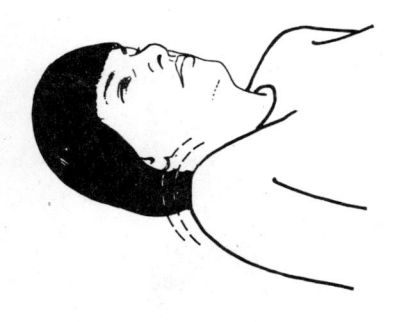

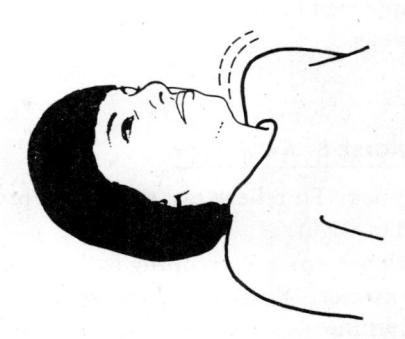

EXERCISE 6: *Tip-toe walking*.

PURPOSE: To strengthen the feet and calf muscles, and develop good posture.
STARTING POSITION: Standing, shoes off.
MOVEMENT: Raise the heels off the floor and walk on the tips of the toes. Walk 100 steps.

Note: Keep the heels raised as high as possible.

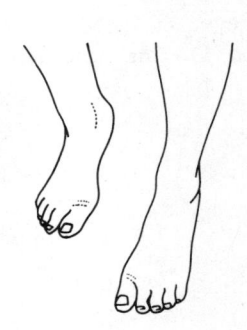

CHINESE FITNESS EXERCISES

EXERCISE 7: *Edge walking.*

PURPOSE: To prevent flat feet, and strengthen the ankle joints.

Caution: This exercise is not suitable for children with ankle problems resulting from injuries to the lateral ligament.

STARTING POSITION: Standing, shoes off.

MOVEMENT: Walk with the feet pointing forward, but with the insides of the feet off the floor (walking on the "edge"). All body weight is supported by the outsides of the feet. Walk 100 steps.

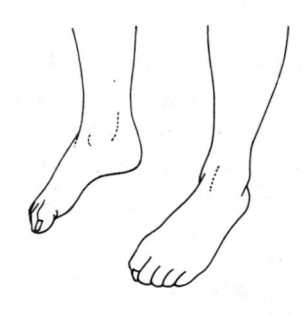

EXERCISE 8: *Eye massage.*

PURPOSE: To relieve eye strain and promote good eyesight.

STARTING POSITION: Sitting with eyes closed.

MOVEMENT: Stroke and press the region around the eyes in a circular motion with the index and middle fingers of both hands, left hand for the left eye and right hand for the right eye.

Note: Do this massage with clean hands.

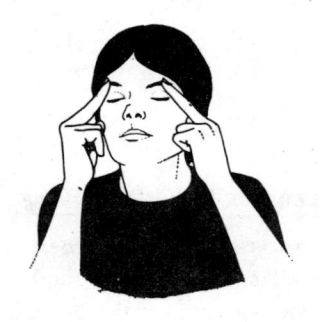

CHAPTER VIII

Fitness Exercises for the Sedentary

Sedentary people should take an exercise break at least once a day in order to keep fit and avoid degenerative conditions such as coronary heart disease and degenerative musculoskeletal problems. The following program is designed to meet such a need. It may be done during an exercise break at work or at home.

CHINESE FITNESS EXERCISES

EXERCISE 1: *Swinging the arms.*

PURPOSE: To improve digestion, blood circulation, and general well-being, and to keep the shoulder joints in good shape and prevent "frozen shoulders."

STARTING POSITION: Standing with the feet shoulder width apart. The trunk is straight, head erect but relaxed, mouth closed naturally, the tip of the tongue placed against the hard palate, eyes looking forward. Arms hang naturally at the sides. Fingers spread naturally.

MOVEMENT: Swing both arms forward and upward as high as the navel. Then swing them downward and backward naturally. With the continuing, rhythmic swinging of both arms, the lumbar region and the pelvis sway forward and backward with the same rhythm. Repeat this swinging motion 100–200 times (about 2–4 minutes), initially. Later, as the level of fitness improves, the number of swinging motions may be increased to 300–500.

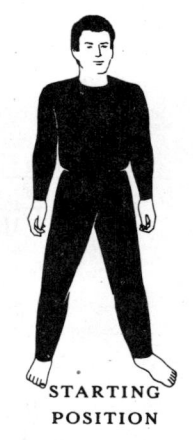

Note: 1. Relax the entire body as much as possible during the exercise. 2. The swinging motion should be light, rhythmic, and effortless, performed at an easy and comfortable rate, about 50 swings per minute. 3. Continue to breathe naturally during the exercise.

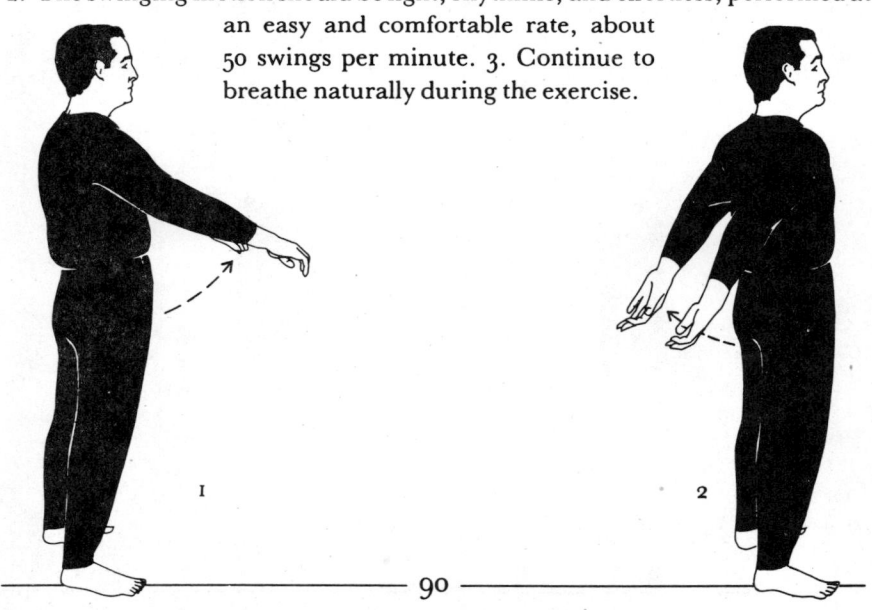

Fitness Exercises for the Sedentary

EXERCISE 2: *Twisting the trunk and looking backward.*

PURPOSE: To develop flexibility of the spine, and prevent stiff neck.

STARTING POSITION: Stride standing (feet separated slightly more than shoulder width).

MOVEMENT: 1. Twist the trunk and head to the left until the heels of the feet are visible. At the same time swing the left arm to the left and place the right hand on the back of the head. Then return to the starting position. 2. Repeat this movement in reverse, twisting to the right, with the left hand on the back of the head. Then return again to the starting position.

Repeat this exercise 10–20 times.

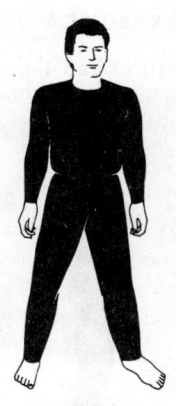

STARTING POSITION

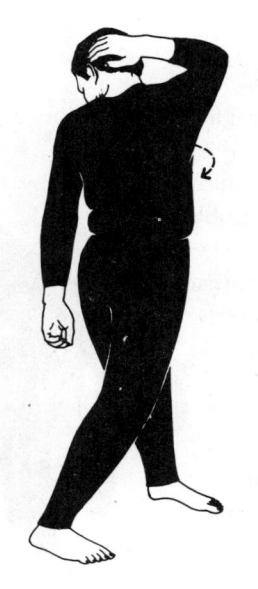

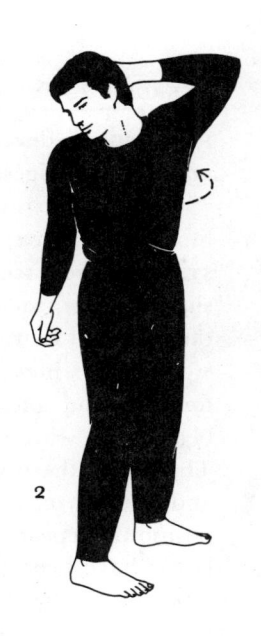

CHINESE FITNESS EXERCISES

EXERCISE 3: *Pushing with the hands while riding a horse.*

PURPOSE: To strengthen the arms and knees.

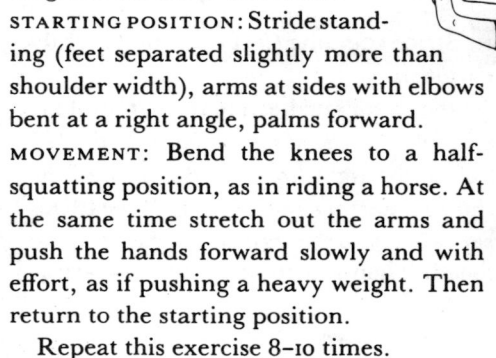

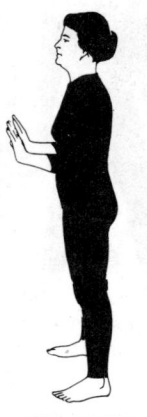

STARTING POSITION: Stride standing (feet separated slightly more than shoulder width), arms at sides with elbows bent at a right angle, palms forward.

MOVEMENT: Bend the knees to a half-squatting position, as in riding a horse. At the same time stretch out the arms and push the hands forward slowly and with effort, as if pushing a heavy weight. Then return to the starting position.

Repeat this exercise 8-10 times.

STARTING POSITION

EXERCISE 4: *Picking up beans.*

PURPOSE: To develop general fitness, flexibility of the spine, and improve digestion.

Caution: This exercise should be avoided by those with lumbar intervertebral disk problems.

STARTING POSITION: Standing with feet slightly apart, 20-50 beans spread over the floor just in front of the feet.

MOVEMENT: Bend the trunk forward and pick up two beans, one with each hand. Then raise the trunk slowly and return to the starting position. Repeat this until all the beans have been picked up off the floor, or until you perspire or feel tired.

STARTING POSITION

Note: Keep the knees straight or nearly straight when bending down.

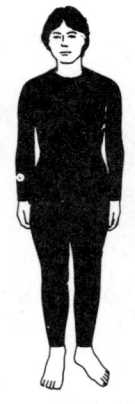

Fitness Exercises for the Sedentary

EXERCISE 5: *Swaying from the waist and hips.*

PURPOSE: To develop flexibility of the lumbar spine and hip joints, and prevent lower back pain.

STARTING POSITION: Standing with feet apart about shoulder width, and hands on hips.

MOVEMENT: 1. Move the pelvis clockwise in a circular motion for 30 seconds. 2. Now, move the pelvis counterclockwise in a circular motion for 30 seconds.

Repeat this exercise 4–6 times.

Note: 1. This exercise should be performed in a relaxed manner. 2. The radius of swaying can be gradually increased.

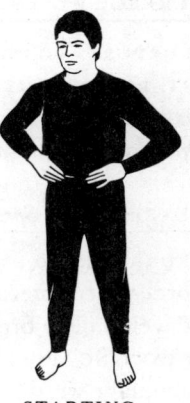

STARTING POSITION

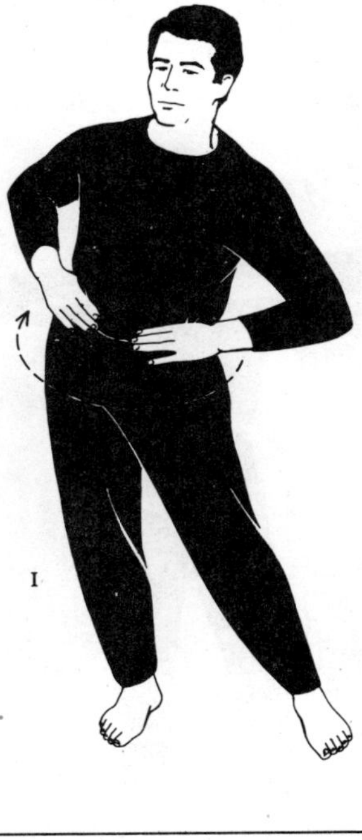

1

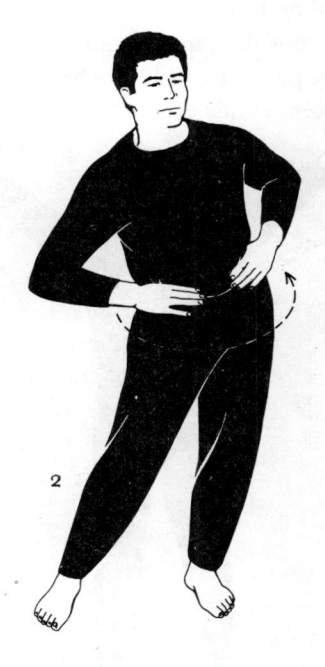

2

TRADITIONAL CHINESE EXERCISES

EXERCISE 6: *Walking like the wind.*

PURPOSE: To improve cardiorespiratory fitness.
STARTING POSITION: Standing.
MOVEMENT: Take a brisk walk. Move as swiftly as the wind, with arms swinging vigorously. Walk for 15–30 minutes.

EXERCISE 7: *Spreading the "wings."*

PURPOSE: To expand the chest and extend the trunk in order to counteract the effects of sedentary posture, and to develop deep breathing.
STARTING POSITION: Standing with feet apart about shoulder width, arms bent at elbows and crossed in front of the chest, palms downward.
MOVEMENT: 1. Extend the elbows and stretch the arms upward and outward. At the same time raise the heels as high as possible, and breathe in deeply. 2. Return to the starting position, and breathe out.
Repeat this exercise 10–20 times.

STARTING POSITION

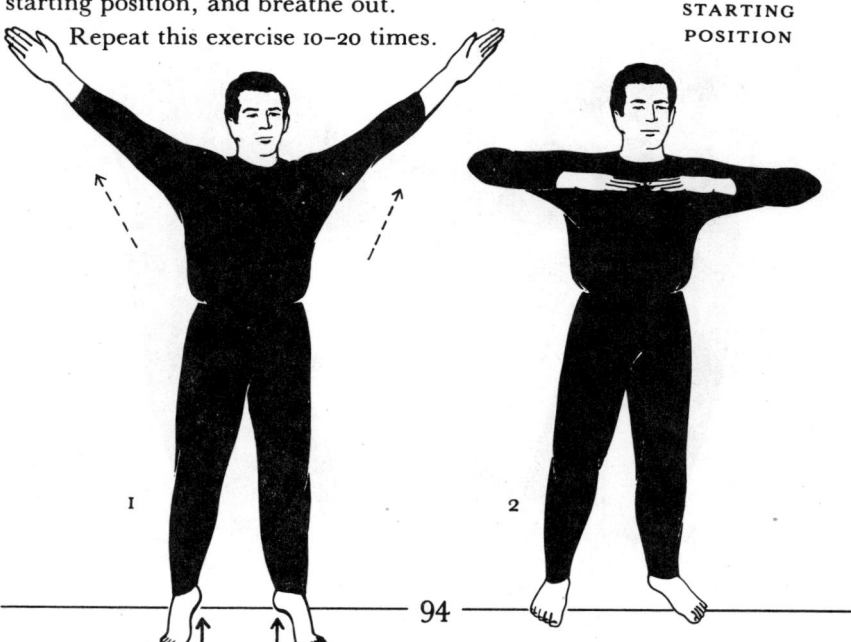

Fitness Exercises for the Sedentary

EXERCISE 8: *Kicking.*

PURPOSE: To stimulate blood circulation in the legs, and develop flexibility of the hip, knee, and ankle joints.
STARTING POSITION: Standing, hands on hips.
MOVEMENT: 1. Lift the right leg and kick forward. Then return to the starting position. 2. Lift the right leg and kick backward. Again, return to the starting position. Repeat this sequence with the left leg.

Repeat the entire exercise 8–10 times.

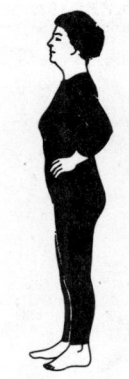

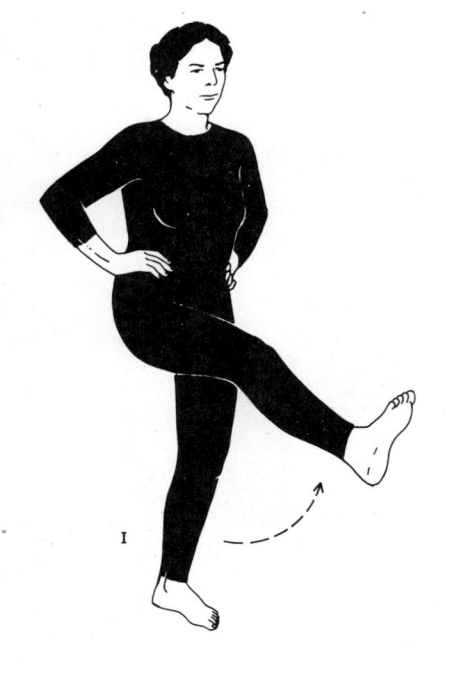

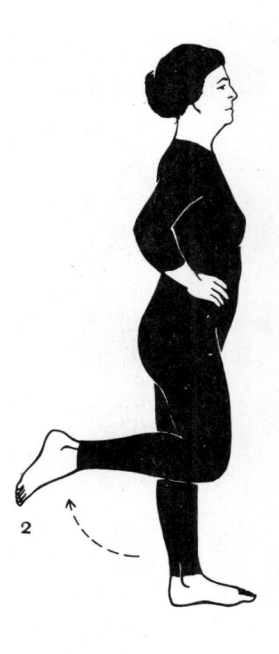

STARTING POSITION

CHAPTER IX

Fitness Exercises for the Elderly

The following program is designed for the elderly with the purpose of improving physical fitness and preventing musculoskeletal problems such as weak feet, backache, and neck pain.

CHINESE FITNESS EXERCISES

EXERCISE 1: *Swinging the arms.*

PURPOSE: To improve digestion, blood circulation, and general well-being, and to keep the shoulder joints in good shape and prevent "frozen shoulders."

STARTING POSITION: Standing with the feet shoulder width apart. The trunk is straight, head erect but relaxed, mouth closed naturally, the tip of the tongue placed against the hard palate, eyes looking forward. Arms hang naturally at the sides. Fingers spread naturally.

MOVEMENT: Swing both arms forward and upward as high as the navel. Then swing them downward and backward naturally. With the continuing, rhythmic swinging of both arms, the lumbar region and the pelvis sway forward and backward with the same rhythm. Repeat this swinging motion 100-200 times (about 2-4 minutes), initially. Later, as the level of fitness improves, the number of swinging motions may be increased to 300-500.

Note: 1. Relax the entire body as much as possible during the exercise. 2. The swinging motion should be light, rhythmic, and effortless, performed at an easy and comfortable rate, about 50 swings per minute. 3. Continue to breathe naturally during the exercise.

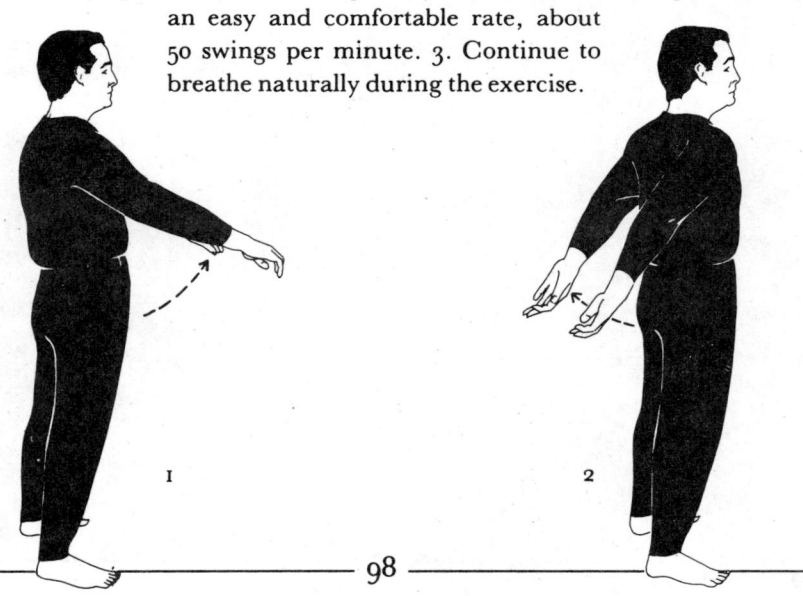

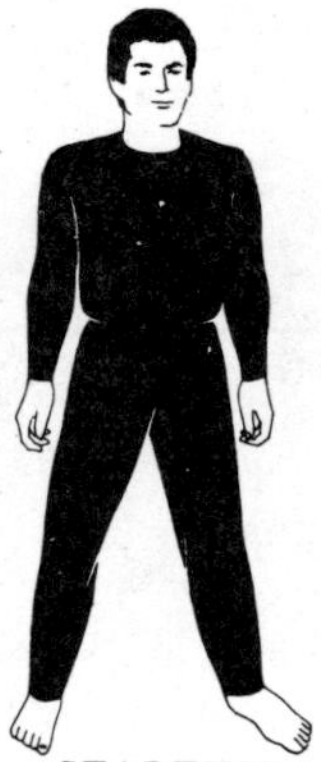

Fitness Exercises for the Elderly

EXERCISE 2: *The cow looking at the moon.*

PURPOSE: To develop flexibility of the neck muscles and cervical spine in order to prevent a stiff neck.

STARTING POSITION: Standing or sitting.

MOVEMENT: 1. Bend the head to the right and twist it slightly up to the left, eyes looking toward the sky (or ceiling). Then return to the starting position. 2. Bend the head to the left and twist it up to the right, eyes looking toward the sky (or ceiling). And again, return to the starting position.

Repeat this exercise 8–10 times.

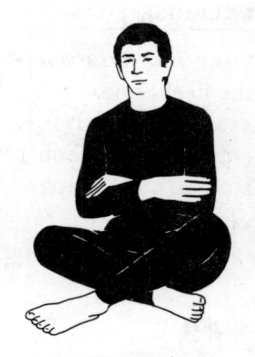

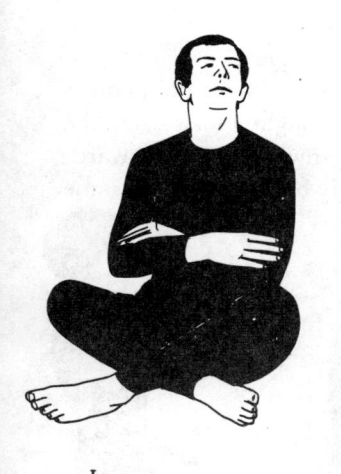

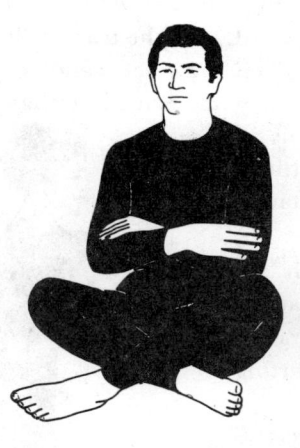

STARTING POSITION

1

2

3

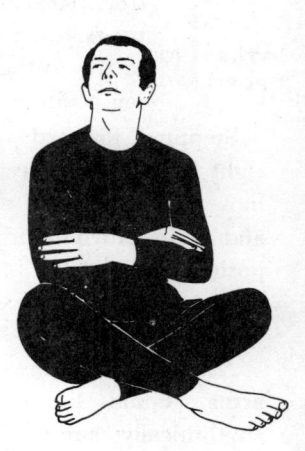

CHINESE FITNESS EXERCISES

EXERCISE 3: *The dragon stamping on the earth.*

PURPOSE: To strengthen the feet and prevent loss of bone mass in the heel bone.

STARTING POSITION: Standing with feet slightly apart. Hands embrace both shoulders.

MOVEMENT: Grip the toes to the ground and stamp with the heels 24 times.

Note: The stamping motion should be moderate in effort.

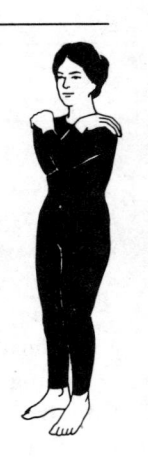

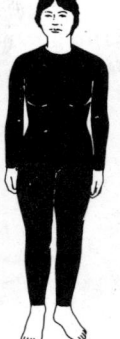

STARTING POSITION

EXERCISE 4: *Rowing.*

PURPOSE: To improve general fitness and develop the flexibility of the spine.

STARTING POSITION: Standing, feet slightly apart.

MOVEMENT: 1. Step forward with the left foot. Stretch both arms forward and upward, with the trunk falling slightly forward at the same time. 2. Then draw the hands downward and backward, with the trunk rising and extending slightly backward at the same time. Repeat this 8 times, then return to the to the starting position.

STARTING POSITION

Stepping forward with the right foot this time, repeat the movements in steps 1 and 2, and again return to the starting position.

Repeat the entire exercise 8 times.

Note: The movement of the arms should be performed rhythmically as in rowing.

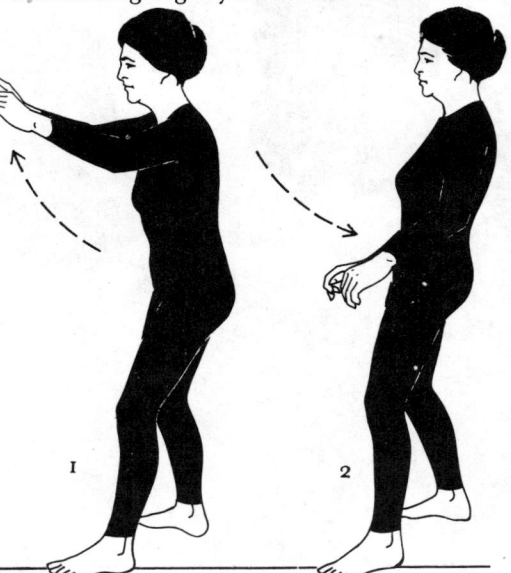

1

2

Fitness Exercises for the Elderly

EXERCISE 5: *Handling two chestnuts with one hand.*

PURPOSE: To facilitate peripheral circulation in the upper arms, and develop flexibility of the finger joints.
STARTING POSITION: Sitting or standing.
MOVEMENT: Place two chestnuts (or small rubber balls, marbles, or smooth round stones) in the palm of the right hand. Move them around with the fingers of the right hand for 2 minutes. Then repeat this using the left hand.

Note: Handle the chestnuts with only one hand at a time, being careful not to let them slip off the palm.

EXERCISE 6: *Half-squatting.*

PURPOSE: To develop flexibility of the hip and knee joints, and strengthen the legs.
STARTING POSITION: Standing, arms at sides.
MOVEMENT: Take a step to the left with the left foot, while bending the knees and hips to lower the body to a half-squatting position. At the same time, bend the elbows and press the hands downward. Then return to the starting position. Repeat the movement, this time stepping to the right. Then return again to the starting position.

Repeat the entire exercise 8–10 times.

Note: Do the half-squatting in a relaxed manner.

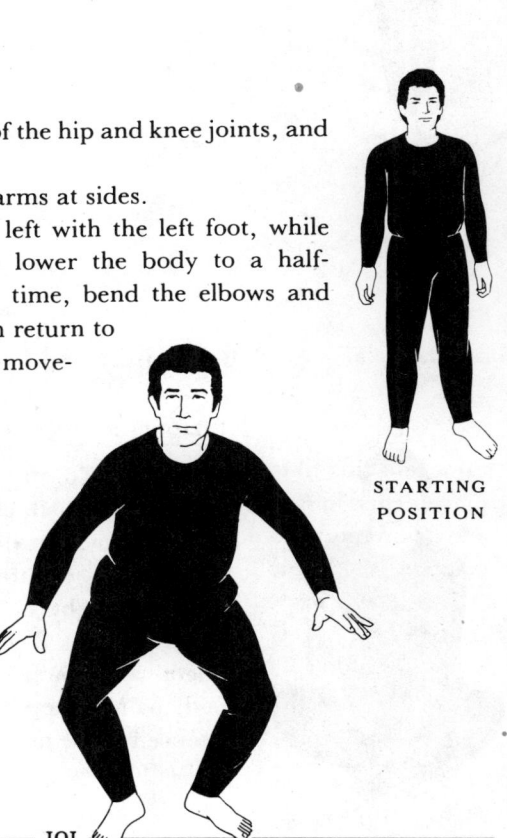

STARTING POSITION

CHINESE FITNESS EXERCISES

EXERCISE 7: *Walking and massaging the abdomen.*

PURPOSE: To stimulate digestion and blood circulation, especially after having a big meal.
STARTING POSITION: Standing.
MOVEMENT: Walk 100–500 steps at a comfortable pace. Meanwhile, massage the abdomen with both hands in a circular stroking manner.

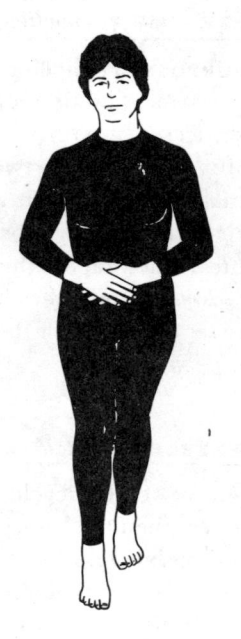

STARTING POSITION

Self-administered preventive massage

1. *Hitting the arms and legs.*

PURPOSE: To stimulate peripheral blood circulation.
STARTING POSITION: Sitting.
MASSAGE: 1. Hit the left arm with the right open hand, then reverse. 2. Then slap the thighs and lower legs with both palms. Repeat this sequence for one minute.

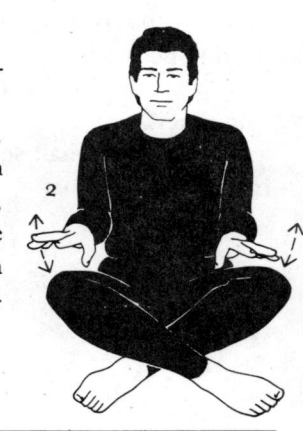

Fitness Exercises for the Elderly

2. *Acupressure on* chu san li *(the point of longevity).*

PURPOSE: To improve general health and strengthen the legs.

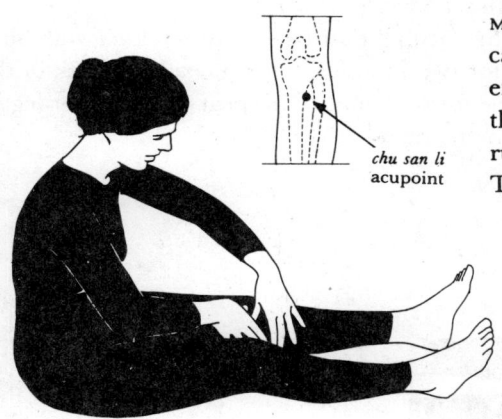

chu san li acupoint

STARTING POSITION: Sitting.
MASSAGE: 1. *Chu san li* is located 2½ inches below the outer edge of the knee cap. Press the point with the thumb and rub it gently for one minute. Then repeat on the other leg.

3. *Stroking the point* shen shu.

PURPOSE: To prevent backache and increase vitality.
STARTING POSITION: Sitting.
MASSAGE: *Shen shu* is located in the lumbar region. Rub or stroke this area for 3–5 minutes.

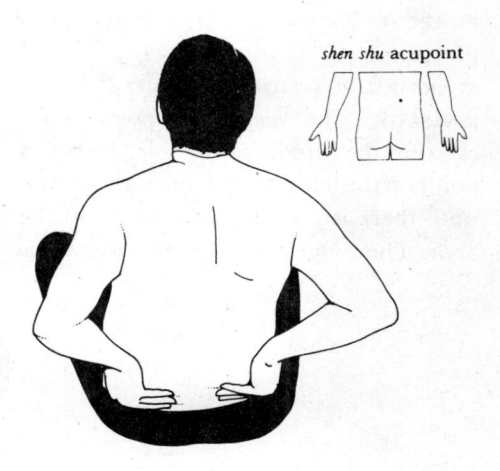

shen shu acupoint

CHINESE FITNESS EXERCISES

4. *Rubbing the knees.*

PURPOSE: To strengthen the knees.
STARTING POSITION: Sitting.
MASSAGE: Rub the surface of the left knee with both hands for two minutes. Then knead the back of the left knee for one minute. Repeat on the other leg in the same manner.

5. *Stroking the point* yung chuan.

PURPOSE: To strengthen the feet, induce sound sleep, and lower high blood pressure.
STARTING POSITION: Sitting.
MASSAGE: The *yung chuan* point is located in the middle of the sole. Rub this point on the left sole with the right thumb until there is a feeling of warmth in the area. Then repeat this on the other foot.

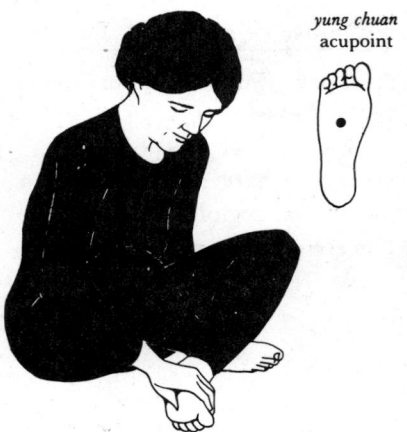

yung chuan acupoint

CHAPTER X

Fitness Exercises for Pregnant Women

Fitness exercises for pregnant women aim to promote relaxation, relieve pelvic pressure, and reduce swelling or edema in the legs. The following program is suitable for the expectant mother from the fourth through eighth month of pregnancy.

CHINESE FITNESS EXERCISES

EXERCISE 1: *Abdominal breathing.*

PURPOSE: To promote relaxation and lift the abdominal wall off the uterus.
STARTING POSITION: Lying on the back, hands on the abdomen, knees bent at about 60°, and feet on the floor.
MOVEMENT: Breathe in slowly protruding the abdomen. Then breathe out slowly, allowing the abdomen to relax.

Repeat this exercise 8-10 times.

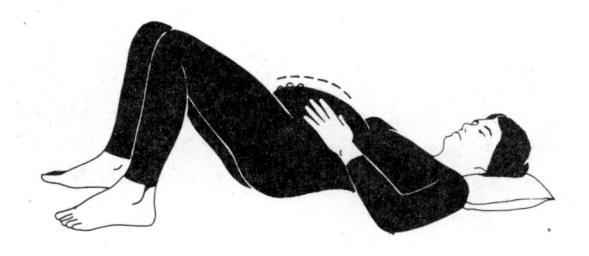

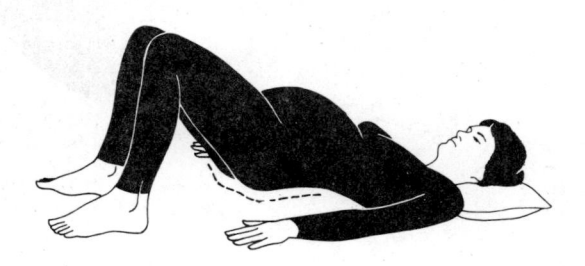

EXERCISE 2: *Pelvic rocking.*

PURPOSE: To prevent or relieve lower back pain.
STARTING POSITION: Lying on the back with knees bent at about 60°, arms at sides resting on the floor, palms down.
MOVEMENT: Raise the buttocks and hips off the floor. Then lower them returning to the starting position.

Repeat this exercise 8-10 times.

Fitness Exercises for Pregnant Women

EXERCISE 3: *Knee bending and relaxing.*

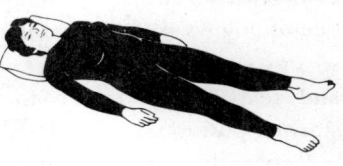

PURPOSE: To help relax the muscles of the pelvic floor.

STARTING POSITION: Lying on the back with legs extended, arms at sides resting on the floor.

STARTING POSITION

MOVEMENT: 1. Bend the knees with the feet moving on the floor back toward the buttocks.
2. Then spread the knees apart, with the soles of the feet touching each other. Relax in this position for a short while.
3. Extend the legs and return to the starting position.

Repeat this exercise 8–10 times.

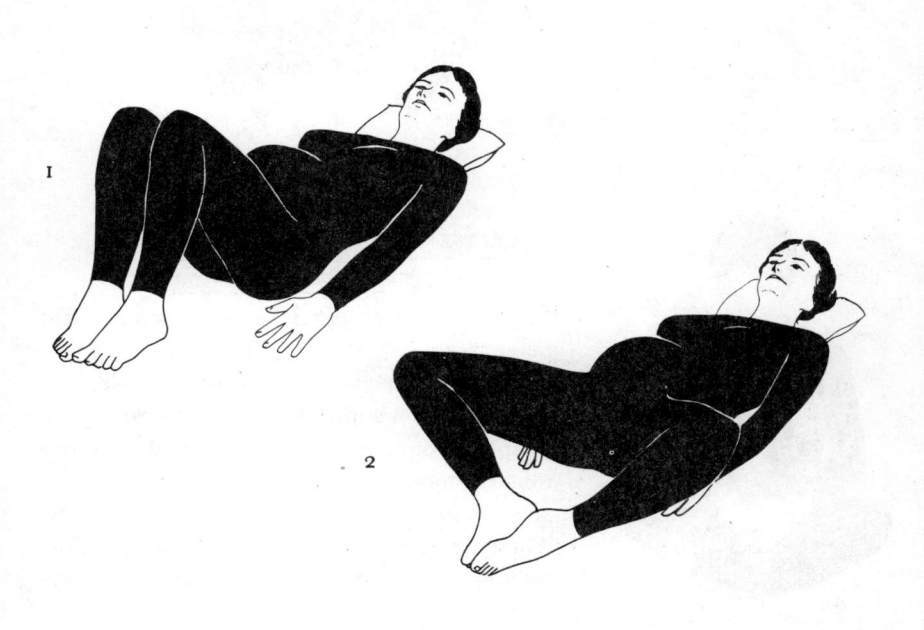

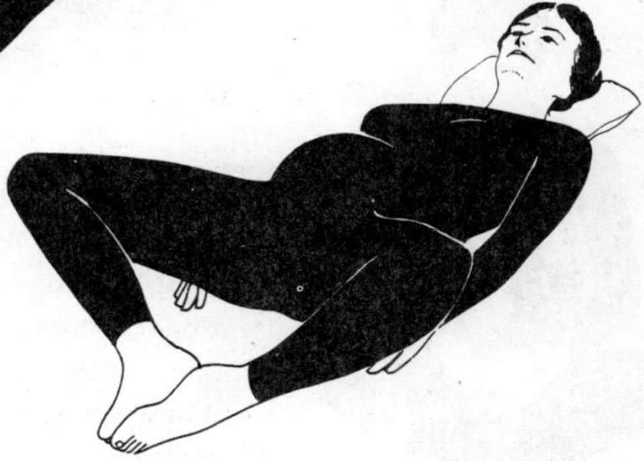

CHINESE FITNESS EXERCISES

EXERCISE 4: *Half-sitting and relaxing.*

PURPOSE: To help relax the muscles of the pelvic floor.
STARTING POSITION: Half-sitting, leaning back against a pile of pillows, knees separated, feet touching the floor.
MOVEMENT: Open the knees wide with the help of the hands, and relax. Then return to the starting position.

Repeat this exercise 8–10 times.

STARTING POSITION

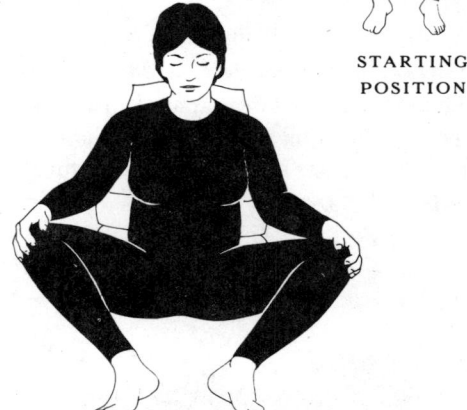

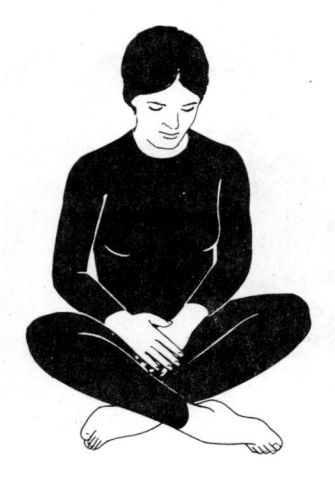

EXERCISE 5: *Tailor sitting (sitting cross-legged) and rhythmic breathing.*

PURPOSE: To help relax the muscles of the pelvic floor.
STARTING POSITION: Sitting cross-legged, with a cushion supporting the buttocks, hands clasped and placed on the lower abdomen in a relaxed manner.
MOVEMENT: Breathe in slowly and naturally. Then breathe out in the same manner, slightly moving the lower back to help relax the hips and buttocks.

Repeat this exercise 8–10 times.

Fitness Exercises for Pregnant Women

EXERCISE 6: *Squatting and relaxing.*

PURPOSE: To help relax the pelvic floor.
STARTING POSITION: Standing with feet shoulder width apart.
MOVEMENT: 1. Bend the knees and take a squatting position with hands resting on the knees. 2. Raise the trunk and return to the starting position with the help of the hands.

Repeat this exercise 6–8 times.

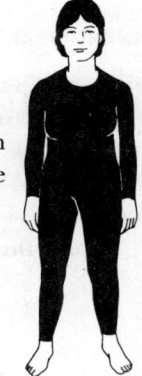

STARTING POSITION

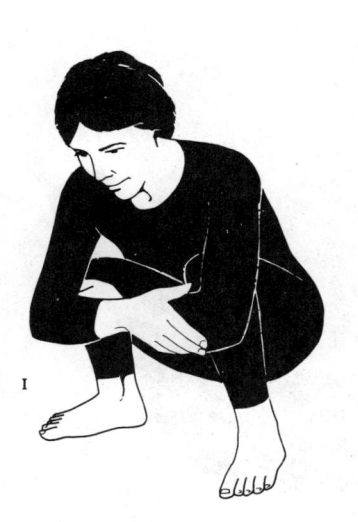

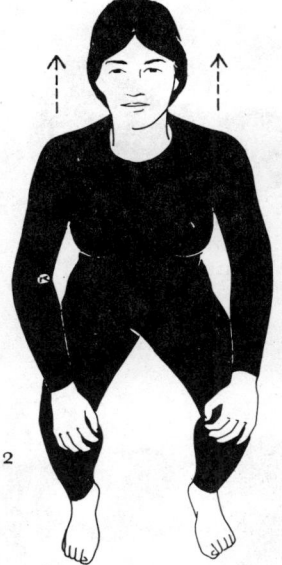

EXERCISE 7: *Walking.*

PURPOSE: To improve blood circulation and digestion.
MOVEMENT: Walk indoors, or, weather permitting, outdoors at a slow and comfortable pace for 5–10 minutes.

CHINESE FITNESS EXERCISES

EXERCISE 8: *Stretching and relaxing.*

PURPOSE: To rest the legs and reduce swelling or edema.

STARTING POSITION: Lying on the back, arms at sides, legs bent, feet pointing at a wall.

MOVEMENT: Raise the legs and place the heels on the wall. Hold this position for one or two minutes. Then return to the starting position.

Repeat this exercise 3–5 times.

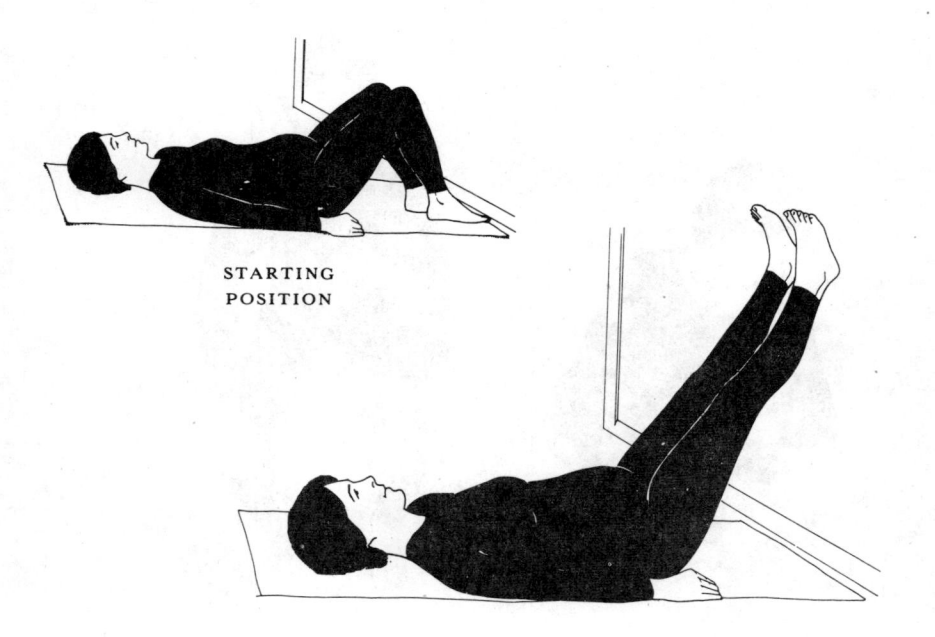

STARTING POSITION

CHAPTER XI

Fitness Exercises for Athletes

The following program is planned for athletes to practice regularly in order to develop the back and knees, and to increase flexibility. It is designed to help in the prevention of sports injuries. When this program is followed after training workouts, the exercises and self-administered massage will facilitate the body's recovery.

CHINESE FITNESS EXERCISES

EXERCISE 1: *Riding a horse.*

PURPOSE: To develop the quadriceps and knees for the prevention of painful knees.

STARTING POSITION: Stride standing (feet pointing forward and separated more than shoulder width), trunk erect, elbows bent at the sides, fists clenched, and toes firmly touching the floor.

MOVEMENT: 1. Bend the knees, as if riding a horse, with thighs parallel to the ground. Hold this position for 2-3 minutes. Meanwhile, take deep breaths. 2. Return to the starting position. 3. Again, bend the knees as in riding a horse. Hold this position for 3 minutes. Meanwhile, stretch out and draw in the arms 6-8 times. When stretching out the arms, do it as if hitting a target with the fists. Then return again to the starting position. This exercise is to be done once or twice only.

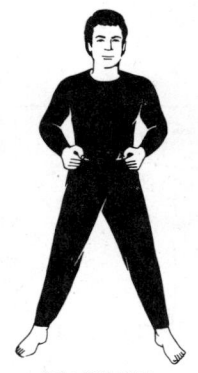

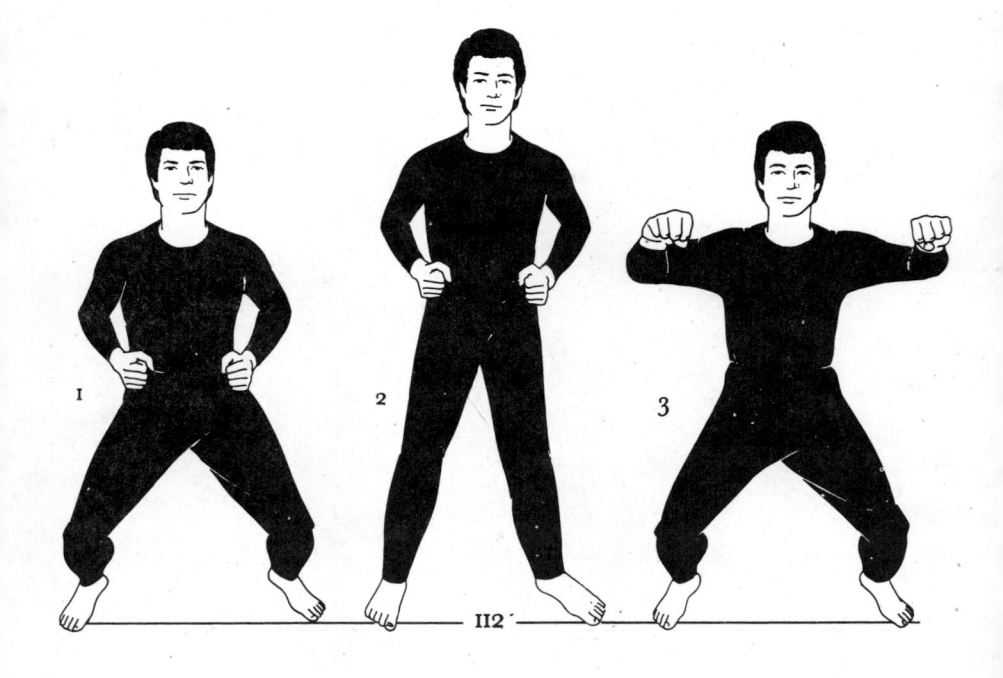

STARTING POSITION

Fitness Exercises for Athletes

EXERCISE 2: *Tiger walking.*

PURPOSE: To develop the flexibility of the lower spine and hip joints.

Caution: This exercise is not suitable for those with back injuries.

STARTING POSITION: Standing with feet separated shoulder width.

MOVEMENT: 1. Bend the trunk forward, bending the knees so the back is almost parallel to the floor. Grasp the left ankle with the left hand, and the right ankle with the right hand. 2. Take a step forward with the right foot, while turning the head to the right. 3. Then take a step forward with the left foot, while turning the head to the left. Walk 8 steps in this manner. Then raise the trunk and return to the starting position. Breathe naturally in a rhythmic manner 8–10 times.

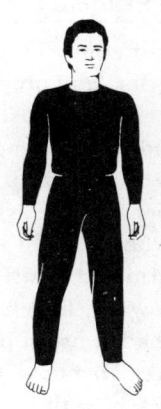

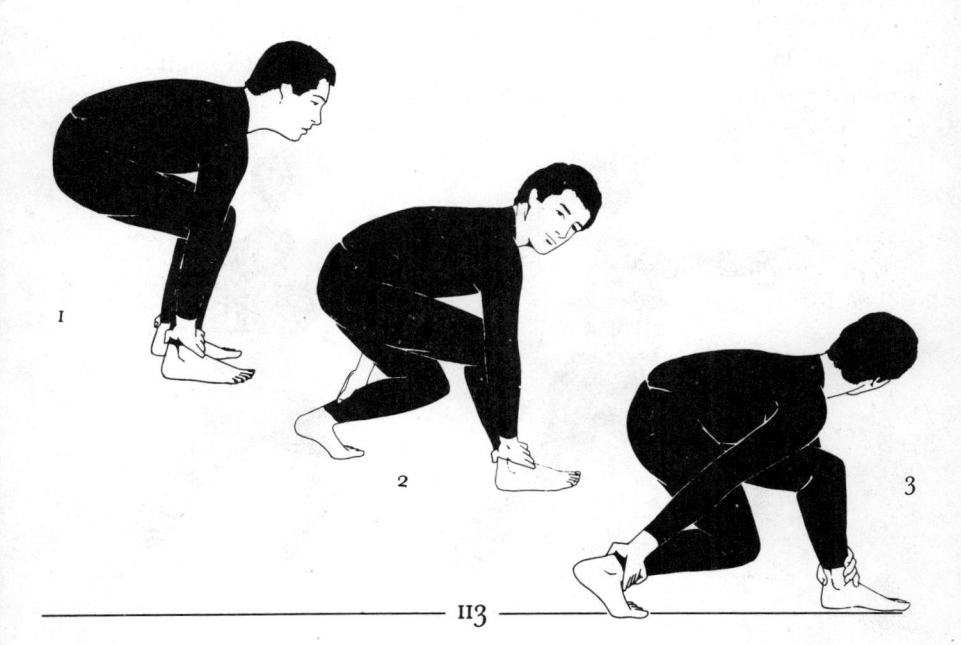

Repeat this exercise 2–4 times.

STARTING POSITION

EXERCISE 3: *Forward thrust.*

PURPOSE: To develop the thighs and hips, the shoulders and arms, and prevent lower back pain.

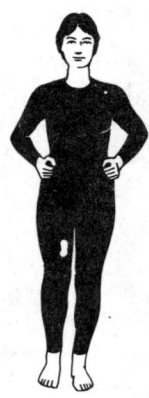

STARTING POSITION: Standing with feet together, arms bent at sides, fists clenched firmly at the waist.

MOVEMENT: 1. Take a big step forward with the left foot, bending the left knee, while keeping the right foot in place, with the right knee straight. Meanwhile, stretch out the right arm and thrust the open hand forward with effort, palm facing inward, fingers together and pointing forward, while keeping the left fist in place. 2. Take a big step forward with the right foot, bending the right knee, while keeping the left foot in place, with the left knee straight. Meanwhile, stretch out the left arm and thrust the open hand straight forward with effort, palm facing inward, fingers together and pointing forward, while drawing in the right hand, fist clenched, to the side of the waist. Continue stepping forward in the manner described above for three minutes (about 100 steps).

Note: 1. Keep the back and head straight during the entire course of the exercise. 2. The knee of the leg which is behind must be kept straight. 3. The forward thrust of the hand should be forceful.

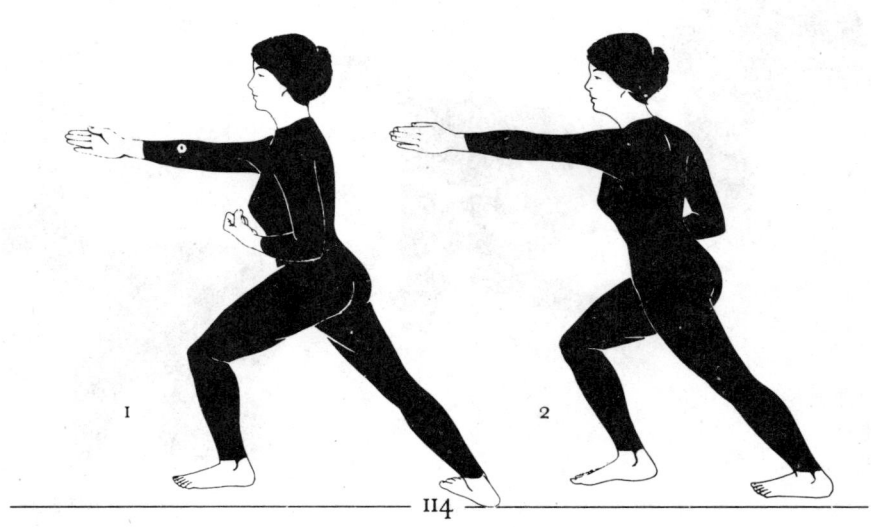

EXERCISE 4: *Swallow flying*.

PURPOSE: To develop the back muscles for the prevention of backache. This exercise is particularly appropriate before a workout.
STARTING POSITION: Lying on the stomach, arms at sides.
MOVEMENT: Raise the head, chest, and legs off the floor simultaneously, with arms swinging backward to assist the trunk movement. Then return to the starting position by dropping the head, chest, and legs to the floor.

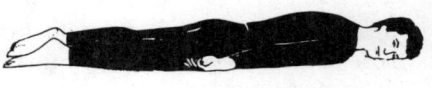

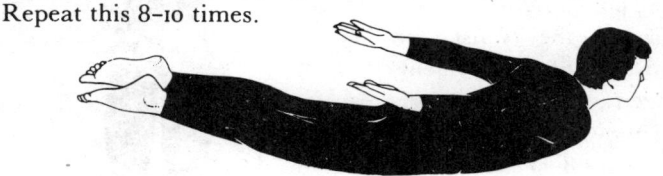

Repeat this 8–10 times.

EXERCISE 5: *Wall pushing*.

PURPOSE: To develop the abdomen and the legs, and strengthen the knees.
STARTING POSITION: Standing with the back against a wall.
MOVEMENT: Bend the knees and move the feet out to lower the body to a half-squatting position with thighs parallel to the floor. In this position, push the back against the wall by pushing with the legs as hard as possible, and hold for five seconds. Then rest five seconds in the half-squatting position. Finally, return to the starting position.

Repeat this exercise 2–4 times.

Note: Hands should not press on the thighs at all.

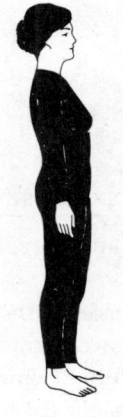

CHINESE FITNESS EXERCISES

EXERCISE 6: *Hanging and swinging.*

PURPOSE: To relieve strained back muscles and spine in order to prevent back pain. It is particularly suitable for athletes after a workout.

STARTING POSITION: Standing on toes with feet together. Hands reaching upward as far as possible, grasp an overhead bar in order to stretch the trunk. Elbows and legs are kept straight.

MOVEMENT: 1. Swing the waist ten times in a clockwise circular movement. 2. Then swing it ten times in a counterclockwise circular movement.

Repeat this sequence 8–10 times.

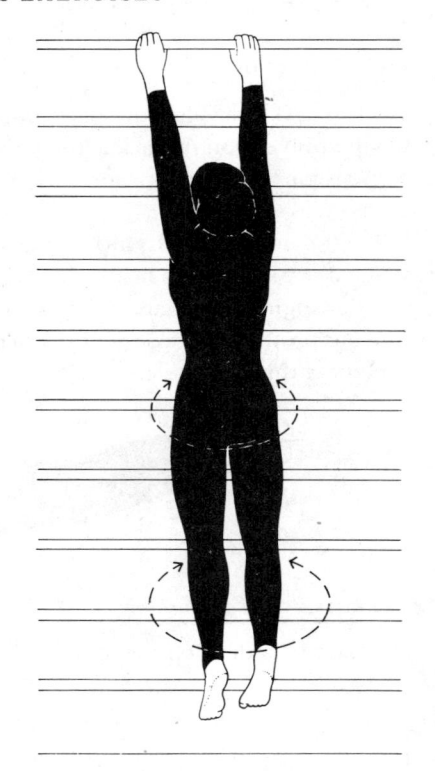

EXERCISE 7: *Relaxing the waist and tapping the body.*

PURPOSE: To aid in relaxing the body.
STARTING POSITION: Standing with feet apart, arms at sides, fists clenched slightly, body relaxed.
MOVEMENT: 1. Twist the trunk to the left, while at the same time swinging the arms easily to the left. Let the swinging right fist hit the left abdomen, and the left fist hit the lower

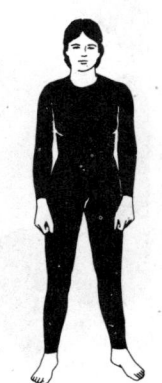

STARTING POSITION

Fitness Exercises for Athletes

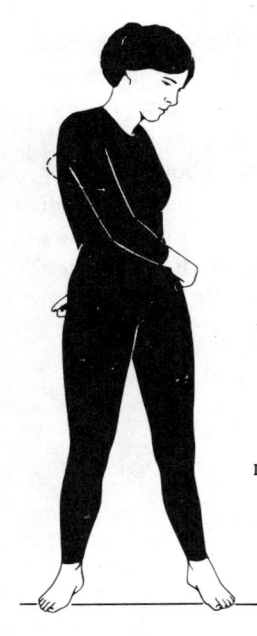

back on the right side. 2. Twist the trunk to the right, while swinging the arms easily to the right. Let the swinging left fist hit the right abdomen, and the right fist hit the lower back on the left side.

Note: The hitting should be moderate in effort.

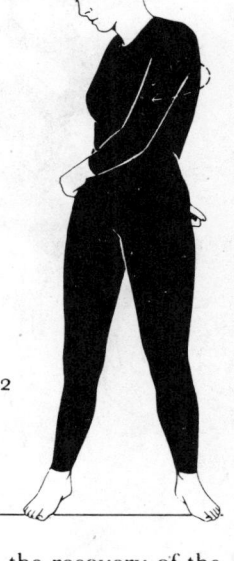

1

2

―――Self-administered massage―――

PURPOSE: To help prevent sports injuries, and facilitate the recovery of the body after a workout.

STARTING POSITION: Sitting on a chair.

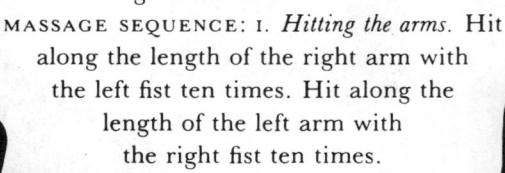

MASSAGE SEQUENCE: 1. *Hitting the arms.* Hit along the length of the right arm with the left fist ten times. Hit along the length of the left arm with the right fist ten times.

2. *Hitting the thighs.* Hit the thighs with both fists 20 times.

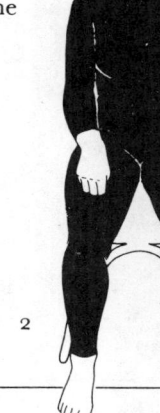

1

2

CHINESE FITNESS EXERCISES

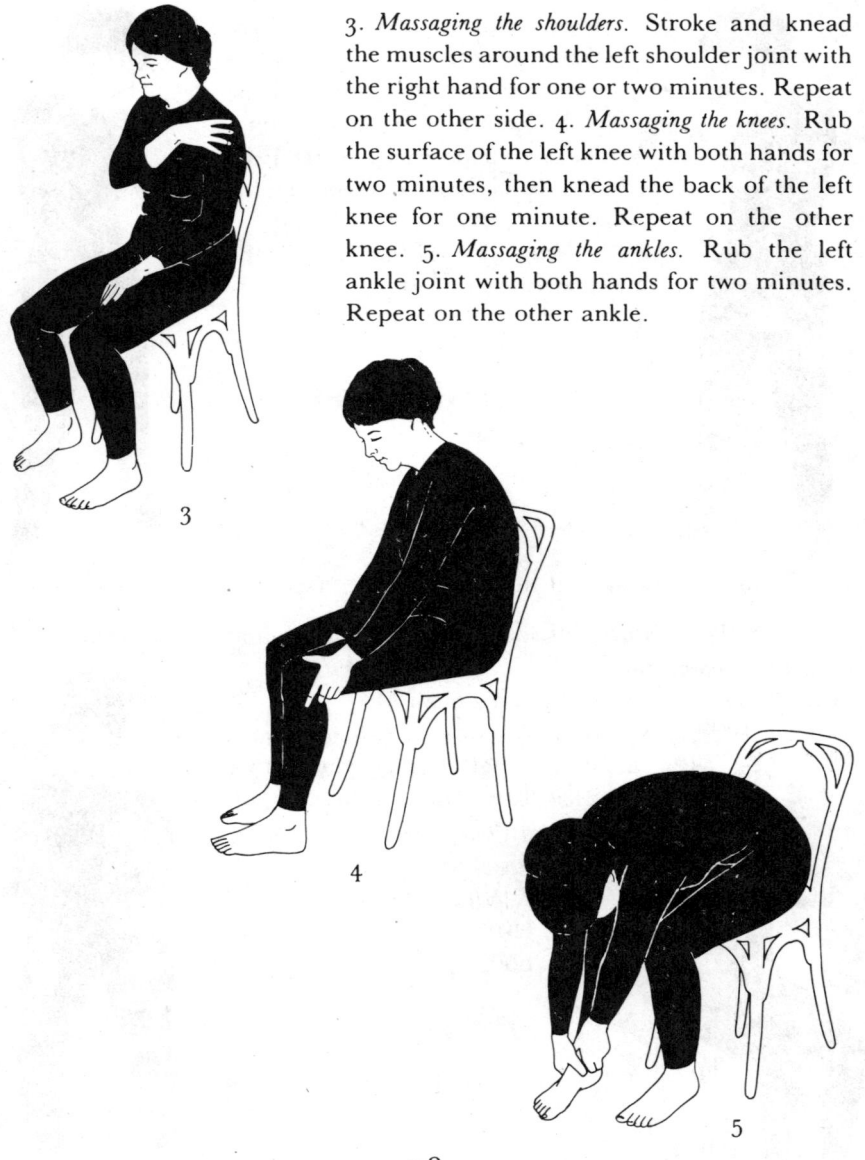

3. *Massaging the shoulders.* Stroke and knead the muscles around the left shoulder joint with the right hand for one or two minutes. Repeat on the other side. 4. *Massaging the knees.* Rub the surface of the left knee with both hands for two minutes, then knead the back of the left knee for one minute. Repeat on the other knee. 5. *Massaging the ankles.* Rub the left ankle joint with both hands for two minutes. Repeat on the other ankle.

PART III
Chinese Therapeutic Exercises

CHAPTER XII

Exercises for Hypertension

Over the past three decades, Chinese exercise therapy has been used in the treatment of hypertension with favorable results. A comprehensive program for hypertension includes such exercises as *Chi Kung, Tai Chi Chuan,* walking, massage, therapeutic exercise, and remedial games. Any one of these can be used alone or along with one or two other forms of exercise therapy. The best combination would be *Chi Kung, Tai Chi Chuan,* massage, walking, and swimming.

It usually takes about three months to obtain significant therapeutic results. These may include lasting reduction in blood pressure, relief of symptoms (such as dizziness, headache, insomnia, palpitation), an increase in efficiency of heart and lungs leading to generally improved physical functioning, as well as the improvement of one's emotional and psychological state.

All the exercises should be performed at a comfortable pace and in a relaxed manner. Hypertensive patients respond to strenuous exercise in a drastic manner, with a sharp rise in blood pressure and heart rate, which may be accompanied by increasing headache and dizziness. In some hypertensive patients, angina—acute chest pain—may be triggered by vigorous exercise. Furthermore, when exposed to contact games, hypertensive patients, who are usually poor in balance and co-ordination, have to face the risk of falls and collisions resulting in internal bleeding. It is therefore important to avoid strenuous exercises and contact games in an exercise program for hypertensive patients.

Chi Kung

The effects of *Chi Kung* in the treatment of hypertension consist of lowering the blood pressure, decreasing the sensitivity of the body to mental stress, and reinforcing the therapeutic effect of hypertensive drugs. To achieve these results, hypertensive patients using *Chi Kung* therapy should try their best to attain relaxation, serenity, and "letting go" (letting the tension go and the blood pressure go down). The most commonly used techniques for this purpose are *Chi Kung for Relaxation* and *Standing Chi Kung*.

Chi Kung for Relaxation: Sitting on a comfortable chair or on a stool, the patient is to breathe naturally and use the cue words "relaxed" and "quiet" to induce a relaxation response. All areas of the body, including the heart and blood vessels, are to be relaxed in this way. (For detailed technique see *Chi Kung for Relaxation,* page 69.)

Standing Chi Kung: The standing posture has already been described in detail in the section, *Chi Kung for Fitness,* page 70. To induce quietness, and relax both mind and body, the patient is encouraged to utilize positive thoughts or imagery as auto-suggestion. For example, one may imagine that fresh rains are falling on the body from the head down to the feet giving a general feeling of freshness, coolness, and relaxation. Or, one may imagine oneself standing in a beautiful garden with fresh air, spring flowers, and other beautiful sights. These pleasant thoughts help the patient relax both mentally and physically, thereby lowering the blood pressure. *Standing Chi Kung* is indicated for those who are moderately fit. If a weak patient cannot stand too long, he may stand for a while and then sit for the remainder of the session. The length of each session starts at 3–5 minutes, then gradually increases to 15–20 minutes. If standing for this length of time cannot be sustained, he or she may rest for a few minutes before resuming the practice.

To achieve a therapeutic effect in hypertension, it appears that *Standing Chi Kung* is superior to *Chi Kung for Relaxation* or to *Chi Kung* in the sitting positions. The reasons for this are two-fold. First, in the standing position, in which the leg muscles are in a state of isometric contraction, the legs are strengthened, enabling the patient to walk at a steadier pace. Standing in that position, combined with steady breathing and auto-suggestion (focusing attention on the lower abdomen or on the soles of the feet), helps conduct blood congested in the region of the head downward. As a result, after a session of *Standing Chi Kung,* the patient will feel the head to be clear and lighter than before, the legs to be stronger, and the walking pace to have become firmer, with better balance. In addition, the standing position itself facilitates reduction in blood pressure. During the practice of *Chi Kung* it is important to observe the principle of descent. By descent is meant the flowing down of the blood and the *Chi* from the head towards the feet. It will be easier to achieve the above effects of descent if the patient practices *Chi Kung* in the standing position with the attention focused on the lower abdomen or on the soles of the feet. It has been shown by experimentation that during a session of *Chi Kung,* infusion of blood in the limbs increases as a result of expansion of the peripheral arteries. It has also been demonstrated that blood pressure drops when attention is focused on the lower abdomen, while it rises when attention is focused on the tip of the nose.

The influence of *Chi Kung* on blood pressure may be accounted for by its action on the autonomic (or "automatic") nervous system which unconsciously controls many of our vital functions. The autonomic nervous system exists in two parts, one speeding up certain physiological processes (such as the heart rate and respiratory rate) and the other slowing them down. It has been observed, in hypertensive patients, that *Chi Kung* therapy changes the balance of these functions, favoring those producing the slow down effects, thus lowering blood pressure by relaxing the muscle around the arteries. Responses to environmental stimuli such as light and sound, and also to internal stimuli such as limb and joint position and movement, are also lessened, thus producing a state of general relaxation that also contributes to reducing hypertension. Animal experiments suggest that a decrease in internal stimuli would result in a reduction in activity of the hypothalamus and visceral sympathetic nerves, and this, in turn, provides a basis for explaining the antihypertensive effect of *Chi Kung.*

Clinical observations have proved that the beneficial effects of *Chi Kung* on hypertension will be reinforced only when the patient keeps up the practice of this exercise. One cannot be satisfied with the transient blood pressure reduction observed at the end of a *Chi Kung* session, as this is simply the immediate result of relaxation and gentle breathing. Radical and lasting improvements in the condition can only be guaranteed by profound alteration in the functioning of the nervous system, which emerges through the long-term practice of *Chi Kung*.

Therapeutic exercise and sports

The best selection of exercises for a hypertensive patient is *Chi Kung, Tai Chi Chuan,* massage, walking, and swimming. Patients with only mild hypertension may take part in jogging as well.

Tai Chi Chuan: Tai Chi Chuan is an excellent exercise for hypertensive patients.

First, the gentle movement and the relaxed stance of *Tai Chi* can reflexively induce the dilatation of the small blood vessels and thus lower the blood pressure. We have observed that a decrease in systolic pressure by 10–15 mmHg was achieved in hypertensive patients immediately after practicing a set of *Tai Chi*.

Secondly, *Tai Chi Chuan* is a mental exercise which requires that the participant become concentrated and peaceful in mind — a good remedy for the distractedness and mental hypersensitivity seen in many hypertensive patients.

Thirdly, because many movements in *Tai Chi* are coordinative or balancing in nature, they are useful in improving the balance and coordination of hypertensive patients.

There are two programs of *Tai Chi Chuan* — Simplified *Tai Chi Chuan* and Old Form *Tai Chi Chuan*. It is advisable for the average hypertensive patient to take up Simplified *Tai Chi Chuan,* because it is much easier and less intense than the older form. For those whose physical condition is too poor to complete an entire sequence, individual movements may be selected. We have found some movements of *Tai Chi* to be particularly beneficial for the hypertensive patient. For example, a stretching exercise called "The white crane spreads its wings" and a coordination exercise called "Parting the wild horse's mane on both sides" are each relaxing and gentle enough to produce relaxation in hypertensive patients. They may repeat each movement 8–12 times and should benefit equally from these exercises. (See pages 23–24.)

Exercises for Hypertension

Therapeutic exercise: The program of therapeutic exercise for hypertensive patients consists of a breathing exercise, relaxation exercise, head movement, stretching exercises of the limbs and trunk, and simple and complex walking. It should be practiced 2-3 times daily, 20-30 minutes for each session, either in class or individually.

Breathing exercise.

STARTING POSITION: Sitting on a chair, hands on thighs.
MOVEMENT: 1. Breathe in slowly and naturally. 2. Breathe out slowly and naturally.
Repeat this 6-8 times.

Relaxation exercise.

STARTING POSITION: Standing with feet apart shoulder width.
MOVEMENT: Swing the arms forward and backward, one moving forward while the other goes back. With the continuing, rhythmic swinging of the arms, swaying the lower back and pelvis forward and backward with the same rhythm.
Repeat the swinging motion 100 times (for about 2-3 minutes).

STARTING POSITION

─────────── CHINESE THERAPEUTIC EXERCISES ───────────

Head exercise.

STARTING POSITION: Sitting on a chair.
MOVEMENT: 1. Bend the head forward, then extend the head backward. 2. Tilt the head to the left, then to the right. 3. Turn the head to the left, then to the right.

Repeat each of the above movements 8–10 times, and then go on to the next.

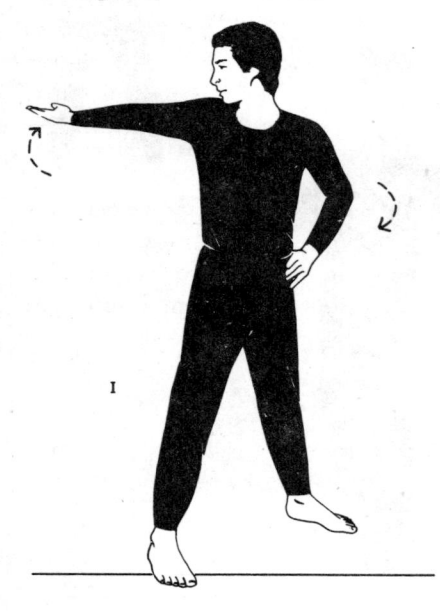

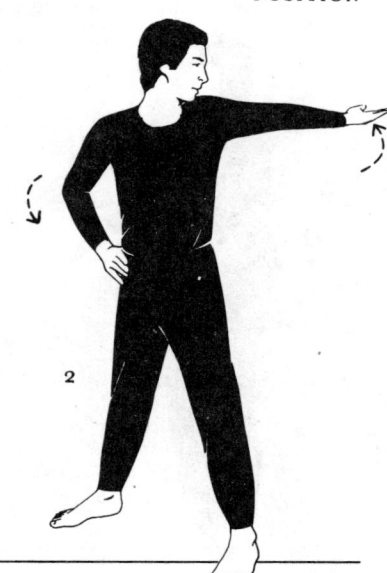

Stretching exercise 1: Sideward stretch.

STARTING POSITION: Standing, feet apart shoulder width, hands on hips.
MOVEMENT: 1. Twist the trunk to the left and stretch the left arm horizontally backward, elbow straight, palm upward. Then return to the starting position. 2. Twist the trunk to the right and stretch the right arm horizontally backward, elbow straight, palm upward. And again, return to the starting position.

Repeat this 8–10 times.

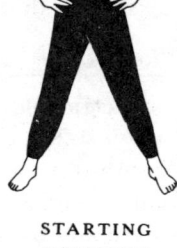

STARTING POSITION

1

2

Stretching exercise 2: Upward stretch.

STARTING POSITION: Standing, feet together, arms at sides.
MOVEMENT: 1. Take a step forward with the left foot and stretch both arms forward and upward. And return to the starting position. 2. Take a step forward with the right foot and stretch both arms forward and upward. Again, return to the starting position.
Repeat this 8–10 times.

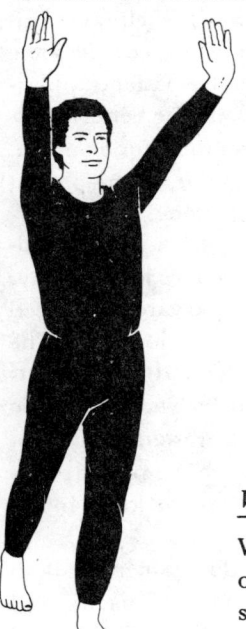

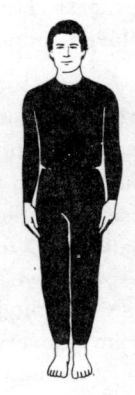

STARTING POSITION

Walking.

Walk at various speeds in the therapeutic gymnasium or or in a big room at home. Start with normal speed (80–90 steps per minute) for 3 minutes. This is followed by a brisk walk at a rate of about 110 steps per minute for 2 minutes. Then take a relaxed and slow walk to complete the exercise session.

Walking: It has been reported that walking on level ground for a prolonged period of time will cause a significant decrease in diastolic pressure. In general, walking is practiced in the early morning, in the evening or before going to sleep — once or twice daily, 15 minutes to an hour per session, at moderate speed. On the weekend, the patient may go on a longer journey on foot for sightseeing, or, if not too rigorous, he or she may go hiking in the hills.

Swimming: Patients who have already mastered this skill may swim outdoors on warm and sunny days or indoors in a warm pool. Therapeutic swimming must be practiced in a slow and relaxed manner, and for short distances only.

Games: Hypertensive patients may benefit from games that are simple, relaxed, non-competitive, and of low intensity.

Jogging: Jogging, properly prescribed and executed, may be helpful to improve the tone of the autonomous nerves. Since jogging may cause some drastic responses in the cardiovascular system of hypertensive patients, physicians should be cautious when prescribing jogging. It would be better to advise the patient to first participate in a brisk walking program, for example, walking ½ to 1 mile (1–2 km) at the rate of 3 miles per hour. If the patient responds well to the brisk walking, he may progress to jogging.

A chronic patient in poor physical condition should begin a jogging program at a very low intensity. One might start with short distance jogging, say, 50 yards, and then increase gradually to 100, 150, and then 200 yards at a speed of 100 yards in 30–40 seconds. Another form of easy jogging is jog/walk. The patient jogs for a short while, then walks for a short while, and then repeats jogging. For example, jogging for 30 seconds followed by walking for 60 seconds, the cycle can be repeated 20–30 times. Such a session would last 30–40 minutes. The speed is generally slow, and adapted to the participant's level of fitness. This form of interval jogging trains the heart at a lower intensity and guards against exhaustion.

Start the program by jogging short distance, and gradually increase both distance and speed. Patients should jog within the limits of their capacity, and stop jogging before they feel exhausted. Never over-stress the heart or exceed the target heart rate prescribed by the physician.

When jogging, breathing should be natural and rhythmic: an inhalation for two steps, then an exhalation for the next two steps, or three steps for each inhalation and exhalation.

It is best to practice jogging in the early morning. However, an afternoon session is acceptable for those who do not have time in the morning. A warm-up of 5 to 10 minutes and a similar cool-down should be included in each jogging session. Participants should be taught to constantly monitor changes in their pulse rate and to watch for other changes of subjective feeling. General health and physical fitness and the suitability of the jogging program should be reassessed regularly by a physician.

Hill climbing: Climbing up a 30–60 yard hill with a slope of 30–40 degrees is indicated for young hypertensives who are fairly fit and have no complications in the early stages of their illness. The climbing is usually done with periods of rest.

Massage

Chinese manipulation and massage: Following a session of *Chi Kung* or therapeutic exercise, a type of sedative massage will be given to the patient as an adjunctive measure to reduce the blood pressure, and to relieve headache and dizziness. For this purpose, the following techniques are commonly used:

Percussion of the head. Tap lightly and quickly on the top of the head or wherever there is discomfort. This is done with the tips of the five fingers.

Kneading the back of the knee (popliteal fossa). Knead the muscles and tendons in the back of each knee with the index, middle, and ring fingers. Knead one knee at a time.

Stroking the point yung chuan. Stroke gently on the point *yung chuan* in the middle of the sole. (See page 64.)

Sedative massage on the head: First, rub both palms to make them warm. Then 1. "Wash" the face with the palms (as in *Shier Duan Jin,* Exercise 3, page 60). 2. Next, stroke the forehead from the midline to both sides with palms and fingers, massaging the occipital region in the same way, and 3. finally, massage the back of the neck and the scapular region.

In a massage session, either or both of the above two techniques may be used. The length of such a massage session should be 5–10 minutes.

CHAPTER XIII

Exercises for Arteriosclerosis

Throughout adult life, the walls of arteries of all sizes become gradually less elastic and more rigid. These changes constitute arteriosclerosis. Chemical analysis has shown that there is also a gradual increase in calcium salts in the arterial walls. These changes alone have little effect on function. However, similar changes, but with some thickening of the arterial walls, are a feature of chronic hypertension. In people with diabetes, the calcific changes may be accelerated and severe. Peripheral circulation may be impaired. In addition, calcific arteriosclerosis is thought to predispose one to another type of arteriosclerosis, namely atherosclerosis, which is by far the most dangerous threat to human life in today's world. Therefore, from a preventive point of view, people with arteriosclerosis should seriously take up an exercise program for both prevention and therapy.

In recent years, a number of investigations have shown that patients with arteriosclerosis may benefit from exercise therapy in the following respects. First, regular exercise may help delay or limit the progression of this disease. It has repeatedly been observed that arteriosclerosis is much milder in laborers and physically active people than in the sedentary, and its severe forms much more common in those who are physically inactive.

Emotional tension and high circulatory lipid (fat) levels are also considered to contribute to the development of arteriosclerosis. Since exercise can relieve tension and can reduce the concentration of lipids in the blood, regular physical training is helpful in preventing the progression of the disease.

As well, exercise can improve blood circulation and relieve symptoms due to peripheral ischemia (deficient blood supply), such as numbness of the hands and feet, and muscular weakness.

Methods of exercise therapy for arteriosclerosis are much the same as for hypertension. In fact, a majority of arteriosclerotic cases are associated with hypertension. The intensity of exercise should be lower in those with severe arteriosclerosis. Typical exercises for arteriosclerotic patients include walking, *Tai Chi Chuan,* therapeutic exercise, and massage. The duration of exercise in one day should not exceed 30–45 minutes.

Walking: Slow walking for 300–1,000 yards on a fine day, preferably in the early morning or in the evening, can stimulate digestion and improve the quality of sleep. Hence walking is a good remedy for insomnia and dyspepsia, which are rather common in patients with arteriosclerosis.

Tai Chi Chuan: As a gentle and soft exercise, *Tai Chi* is particularly good for these patients. They may do the whole set of movements, half a set, or merely some individual movements, depending on their physical condition.

Therapeutic exercise: The goal of therapeutic exercise is to improve the blood circulation of the body in general, and of the limbs in particular. For this purpose, the following exercises and massages were chosen from a program of calisthenics developed in ancient China for the elderly. Preliminary observation of the effects of these modified exercises has indicated that they are of benefit to patients with arteriosclerosis.

EXERCISE 1: Sitting on a chair, clench the fists, and then open the fingers. Repeat this 20 times.

Exercises for Arteriosclerosis

EXERCISE 2: Sitting on a chair, hold two small chestnuts (or small rubber balls, marbles, or smooth round stones) in one hand, and move them around with the fingers of the same hand. Be careful not to let them slip off the palm.

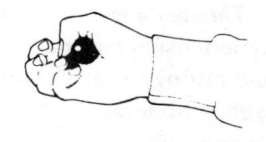

EXERCISE 3: Sitting on a chair, rotate the feet in circles. Repeat this 20 times.

EXERCISE 4: Sitting on a chair, with both hands placed on the back of the neck, 1. twist the trunk to the left, and 2. then to the right. Repeat 20 times. The twisting should be gentle and slow. The number of repetitions for patients with vertigo may be fewer.

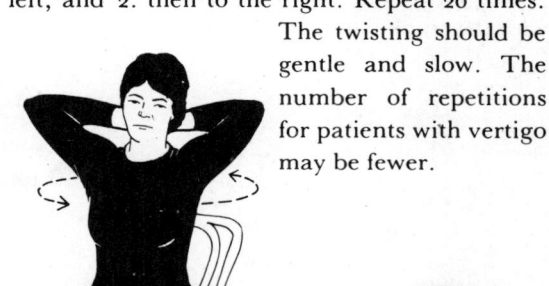

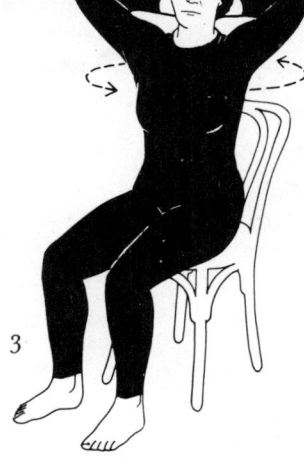

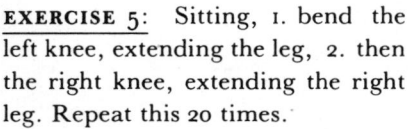

EXERCISE 5: Sitting, 1. bend the left knee, extending the leg, 2. then the right knee, extending the right leg. Repeat this 20 times.

The above exercises may be practiced several times daily.

Therapeutic massage: Sedative massage on the head, neck and shoulder, as for hypertension (see page 129). In addition, slapping the thighs with the palms and hitting the arms with the fists may be done. Such self-administered massage is preferably applied after getting up in the morning, before going to sleep at night, or after therapeutic exercise.

Hitting the arms: Hit the left arm and forearm with the palm of the right fist gently (as in diagram on page 117), then hit the right arm and forearm with the palm of the left fist.

Slapping the legs: Slap the thighs and lower legs with both palms while sitting with the trunk bent slightly forward.

CHAPTER XIV

Exercises for Coronary Heart Disease: Preventive and Therapeutic

Many western visitors to China have been much impressed by the fact that China has a much lower incidence of heart attacks than does the West. Some western physicians have ascribed this to the Chinese way of fitness, namely, doing *Tai Chi Chuan,* jogging, and living a life of moderation. In fact, it is quite true that Chinese exercise plays a part in the prevention and treatment of coronary heart disease.

In terms of the management of coronary heart disease, the strength of the Chinese exercise programs lies in their relaxation-producing effects. Since some types of heart attack and angina are stress-related, a combination of jogging or walking with *Tai Chi Chuan* or *Chi Kung* will result in more effective prevention of heart attack than the use of any of these alone.

Exercise programs presented in this section can be used both for preventive and therapeutic purposes. It is advisable for the patient to have a complete medical evaluation, and to obtain permission from a physician before taking up an exercise program. Once the program is started, general health and physical condition should be reassessed regularly. In addition, the participant in the program should watch carefully for any changes in his or her symptoms and heart rate.

Recent studies suggest that 65–85% of the maximum oxygen intake level is a safe and effective intensity for coronary heart disease patients. That means for a person 50 years of age, a target training heart rate of 110–145 per minute would be desirable. However, one should always remember not to push too hard to reach a target heart rate. It is the level suitable to one's capacity that is important and not a rigid target heart rate. Therefore, during exercise, take a look at the stopwatch from time to time, but do not become its slave.

The other important thing is to integrate exercise with daily life. One should try to use one's legs as much as possible. Again, a preventive life style is essential. Proper diet, adequate physical activity, and control of stress all contribute to the successful prevention and treatment of coronary heart disease.

Coronary heart disease (CHD), also known as coronary artery disease, is a common illness among the middle-aged and elderly. In CHD, the inside of the coronary artery becomes narrow and small, due to the deposit of fat in the inner arterial walls. In addition, the artery tends to be in spasm, reducing the blood supply to the heart muscle, and resulting in deficient blood supply (ischemia) to it. The patient with these pathological changes will suffer from an intense feeling of squeezing pain in the left chest region (angina pectoris). If the involved coronary artery is occluded rapidly, the heart muscle will suffer from acute, severe, and lasting ischemia, and a heart attack will occur.

It appears that lack of physical activity may have something to do with the development of CHD. Studies done in many regions of China have shown that the incidence of CHD in laborers over forty years of age is lower than in sedentary professionals of the same age group. It has been reported that physically active males have a lower incidence of heart attacks as well as a lower rate of mortality within 24 hours of such an attack than do males who are physically inactive. Such findings suggest that regular physical training is helpful in preventing the development of CHD.

Since the 1960's exercise therapy has been utilized with favorable results in treating CHD patients. According to studies done in China as well as in many other countries, exercise therapy may help patients with angina pectoris increase their tolerance for physical activities and improve their physical condition, thus relieving angina. For some patients an improvement in their electrocardiogram was observed. For patients recovering from an acute heart attack, exercise therapy may improve their subjective symptoms, shorten the duration of hospitalization, and increase their physical fitness, thereby promoting vocational rehabilitation.

The mechanisms accounting for the beneficial effects of exercise on CHD may be summarized as follows:

1. Increasing oxygen supply to the heart muscle: Physical activity may stimulate smaller arteries to supply blood to an area where a larger artery is narrowed or closed or it may increase the blood volume in these smaller blood vessels. As a result, blood circulation in the vascular network of the heart muscle may be improved and the oxygen supply to it increased.

2. Reducing oxygen consumption in the heart muscle: Since the adaptation of the blood circulation to exercise is improved by systematic physical exercise, the work of the heart becomes less intense, reducing, to a certain extent, the oxygen consumption in the heart muscle.

3. Improving metabolism of lipids: Experiments have shown that after long periods of physical training, the concentration of cholesterol in the blood is reduced. After eight months of systematic physical training, a steady decline in blood cholesterol levels was seen in a group of middle-aged and elderly people with high blood cholesterol. The improvement in lipid metabolism decreases the deposit of fatty material on the inner walls of the coronary artery.

4. Psychological regulation: Physical activity tends to modify the psychological state of the patient, by producing a more positive outlook and the motivation for maintaining a better lifestyle, as well as removing the preoccupation with CHD. Exercise will ease tension, bringing relaxation and peace of mind, thereby reducing attacks of angina.

5. Promoting fibrinolysis (anti-clotting effect) in the blood: It was reported that exercise of moderate and high intensity had the effect of enhancing fibrinolysis in the blood, thus impeding the progression of atherosclerosis.

There are a variety of exercises suitable for patients with CHD. Apart from the consideration of facilities available, they may choose those which are most suitable to their age, level of health and physical fitness, degree of skill and interest. No matter which exercises they decide upon, the appropriate intensity of the exercise is what counts most. Generally speaking, moderate exercise is preferred.

Walking: A brisk, vigorous walk is more valuable in training the heart than is slow walking. Brisk walking at the rate of 100 steps per minute will increase the heart rate up to more than 100 beats per minute. In brisk walking, it is important to maintain a steady stance and speed, and a smooth rhythm of breathing. If the walking speed is too fast for the body to tolerate, the walker will become breathless, very tired, and even get chest pain. If this occurs, the walking speed should be slowed down. For those for whom walking is their primary means of physical training, the duration of a walking session should be 45–60 minutes, once or twice daily. An alternate schedule is walking 800–2,000 yards a day at normal speed with intermittent sessions of brisk walking.

Jogging: It is recommended that a beginner start by jogging a distance of 50–100 yards, gradually increasing the distance by 100 yards each week. If he or she feels good following such a program, the distance can be increased to 1,000 or 2,000 yards, and, for those at a higher level of physical fitness, even to 3,000 yards.

Terrain cure: This is usually organized in a sanitorium or a large hospital. For those who are fairly weak, a walk of 800–1,000 yards on level ground at a rate of 50–70 yards per minute (i.e., 800–1,000 yards in 15–20 minutes) is recommended. Terrain cure of higher intensity, like the two routes below, may be prescribed for those in better condition.

1. Walking 3,000 yards (level): Walk the first 1,000 yards in 20 minutes, then sit down and rest for 5 minutes. The next 1,000 yards are walked in 16–18 minutes, with another rest, sitting down for 5 more minutes. The last 1,000 yards are to be completed in 20 minutes.

2. Walking 4,000 yards (level) and climbing up a small hill: First, walk 2,000 yards (level) in 40 minutes, then sit down and rest for 5–10 minutes. Follow this by climbing a small hill 30–50 yards high, with a slope of 30–45 degrees, in 30 minutes. After a rest of 5–10 minutes the return journey is resumed at the same rate.

Swimming: Those who have already mastered this skill and are fairly fit may be permitted to take part in swimming. It has been reported that swimming can enhance aerobic capacity in middle-aged people. The increase in oxygen intake after six months of swimming training is similar in effect to the same period of jogging.

Chi Kung: Chi Kung for Relaxation or *Chi Kung for Fitness,* performed in a sitting or lying position, is indicated for CHD patients, especially those undergoing emotional stress or those who are very sick. The following beneficial effects were observed in CHD patients receiving *Chi Kung* therapy: relief from dizziness, improved subjective feeling state, a lifting of depression and more positive general attitude, reduction in the frequency and severity of angina pectoris, and a warm sensation in the hands and feet.

Tai Chi Chuan: As a gentle and relaxed exercise, *Tai Chi Chuan* is suitable for CHD patients with coexisting hypertension or emotional difficulties. It may help lower the blood pressure and remove neurotic symptoms. To increase the degree of exertion, *Tai Chi* may be performed with a lowered stance and large-ranging movements, or else repeated several times in a session.

Comprehensive exercise program: This is generally carried out in a group setting, 2-3 sessions per week, for a half hour to an hour each, preferably scheduled in the afternoon. The content of a comprehensive exercise program includes warm-up, trunk and limb exercises, simple therapeutic sports (such as passing a ball, basketball shooting, bowling, badminton, etc.), walking/jogging, and cool-down. Appendix I (page 141) contains a program used for CHD patients with controlled angina at Zhong Shan Medical College, Guangzhou, China.

Therapeutic exercise: For very sick patients, only simple trunk and limb exercises are prescribed. Avoid any starting position which may elicit angina. For example, if the patient has experienced angina during exercise in a standing position, then he or she is advised to begin a therapeutic exercise program in a lying position. Later, this may gradually be changed to a sitting or standing position, once the patient's condition is improving.

For patients who have recovered from an acute heart attack, simple therapeutic exercises may be prescribed in the initial stage, if the condition is stable. Appendix II contains a program of therapeutic exercise used in the early recovery period for such patients.

Exercises for Coronary Heart Disease

Appendix I
A program of therapeutic exercise for CHD patients
(*Moderate intensity*)

Each of the following exercises is to be repeated 8–12 times unless otherwise indicated.

EXERCISE 1.

Walking at normal speed 1–1½ minutes.

EXERCISE 2.

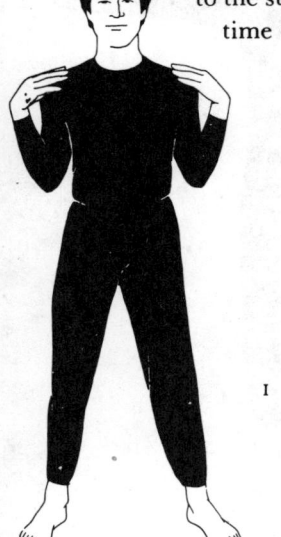

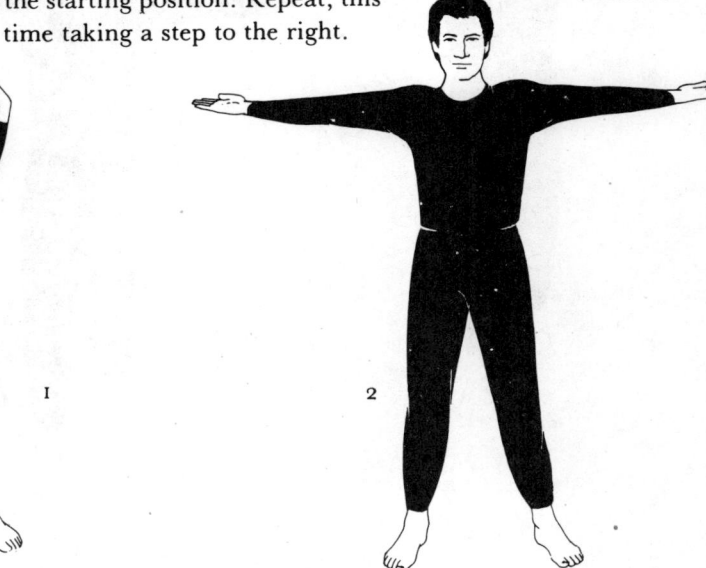

STARTING POSITION: Standing, arms at sides.
MOVEMENT: 1. Take a step to the left with the left foot and bend the elbows at the sides of the body, with fingers touching the tops of the shoulders. 2. Stretch the arms out to the sides at shoulder level, keeping the elbows straight. 3. Bend the elbows back to the sides, fingers touching the shoulders as in step 1. 4. Return to the starting position. Repeat, this time taking a step to the right.

STARTING POSITION

CHINESE THERAPEUTIC EXERCISES

EXERCISE 3.

STARTING POSITION: Standing, arms at sides.
MOVEMENT: 1. Take a step forward with the left foot and bend the elbows at shoulder height so that the fingers meet in front of the chest, palms downward. 2. Stretch the arms out to the sides at shoulder level, elbows straight, palms upward. 3. Bring the arms back with elbows bent as in step 1. 4. Return to the starting position. Repeat, this time stepping forward with the right foot.

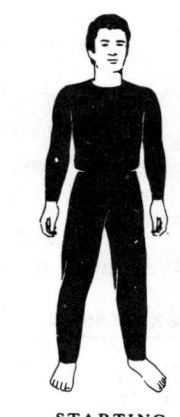

STARTING POSITION

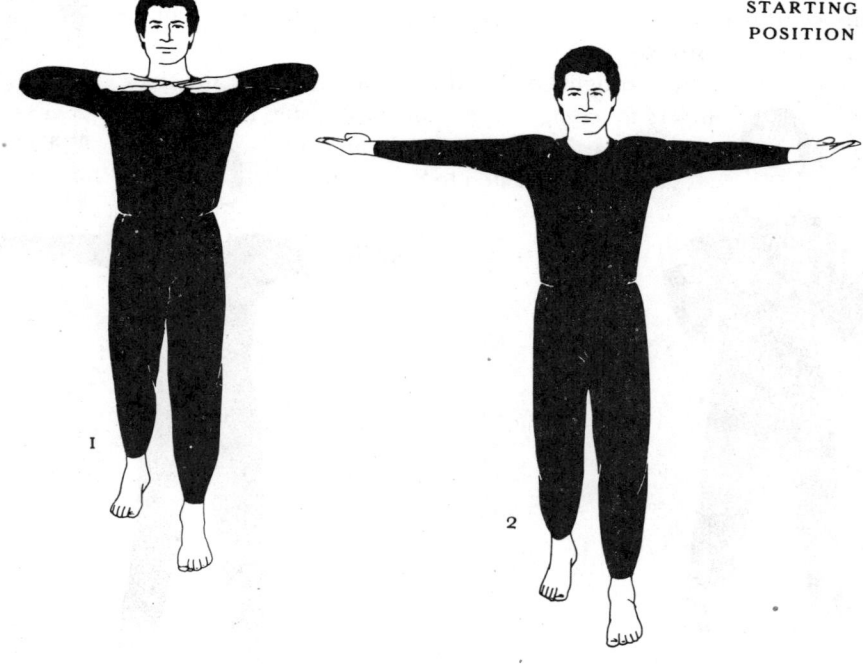

Exercises for Coronary Heart Disease

EXERCISE 4.

STARTING POSITION: Stride standing (feet apart more than shoulder width), hands on hips.

MOVEMENT: 1. Twist the trunk to the left and stretch the left arm back horizontally, elbow straight, palm upward, while the other arm remains on the hip. Then return to the starting position. 2. Twist the trunk to the right and stretch the right arm back horizontally, elbow straight, palm upward. And again, return to the starting position.

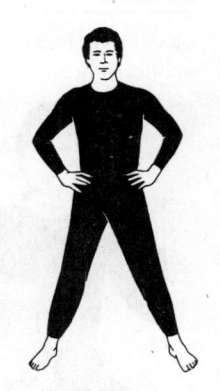

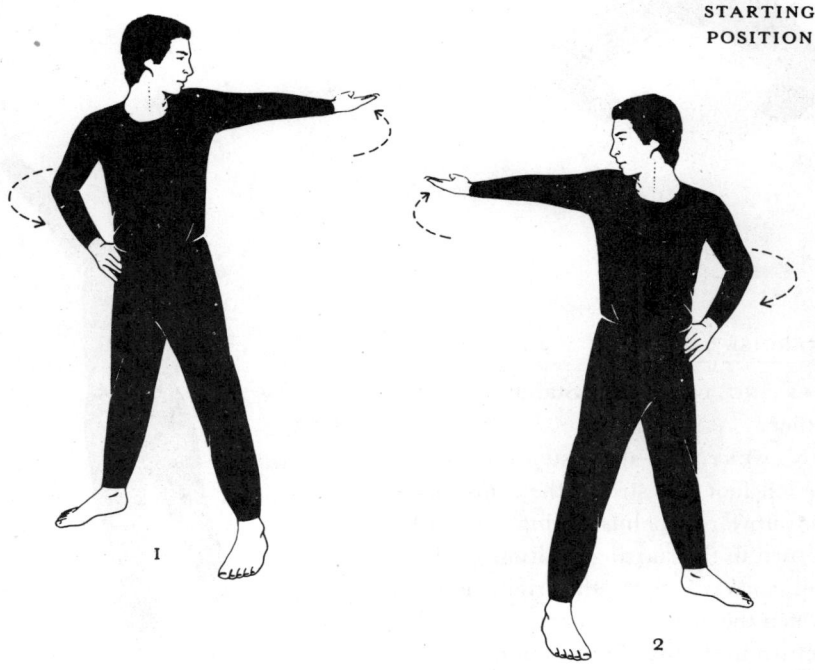

STARTING POSITION

CHINESE THERAPEUTIC EXERCISES

EXERCISE 5.

STARTING POSITION: Standing, feet together.

MOVEMENT: Take a step to the left with the left foot and bend both knees and hips to lower the body. At the same time bend the elbows at sides, fingers touching the top of the shoulders. Then return to the starting position, and repeat the movement, this time stepping to the right.

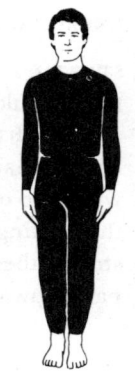

STARTING POSITION

EXERCISE 6.

STARTING POSITION: Standing, feet together.

MOVEMENT: 1. Take a step forward with the left foot and stretch the arms forward and upward, palms facing forward. 2. Return to the starting position. 3. Take a step forward with the right foot and stretch the arms forward and upward. 4. Return to the starting position.

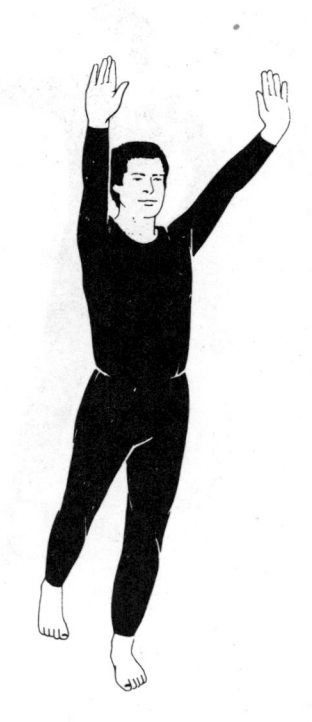

Exercises for Coronary Heart Disease

EXERCISE 7.

STARTING POSITION: Sitting, hands resting on thighs.
MOVEMENT: 1. Bend the head downward, then upward.
2. Turn the head to the left, then to the right.

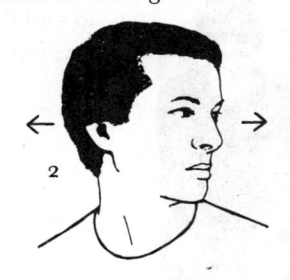

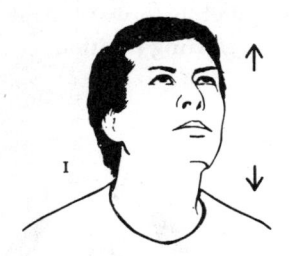

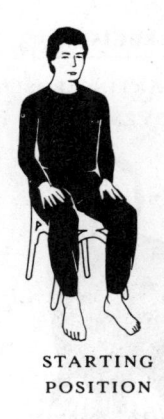

STARTING POSITION

EXERCISE 8.

STARTING POSITION: Sitting, hands resting on thighs.
MOVEMENT: 1. Stretch the arms forward, and then to the sides at shoulder level, palms up, and simultaneously raise the bent left leg. Then return to the starting position. 2. Bring the arms forward and to the sides at shoulder level, palms up, and simultaneously raise the bent right leg. Again, return to the starting position.

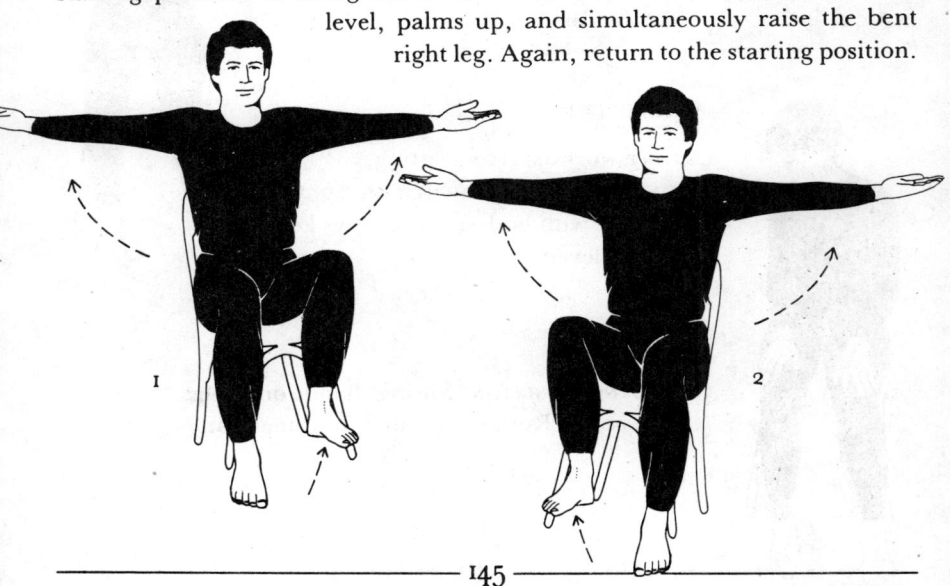

145

CHINESE THERAPEUTIC EXERCISES

EXERCISE 9.

STARTING POSITION. Sitting, keeping hips firm.
MOVEMENT: 1. Bend the head and the trunk slightly backward. Then return to the starting position. 2. Bend the head and the trunk slightly forward. And again, return to the starting position.

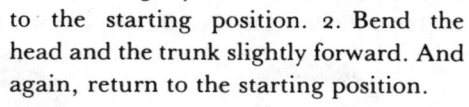

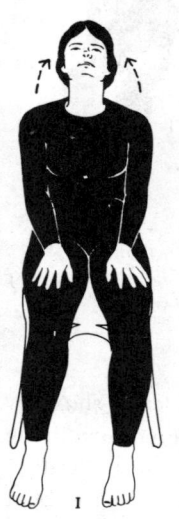

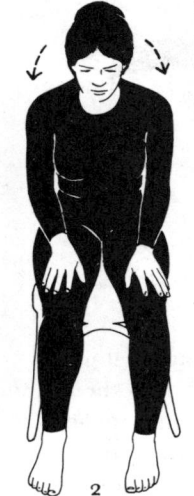

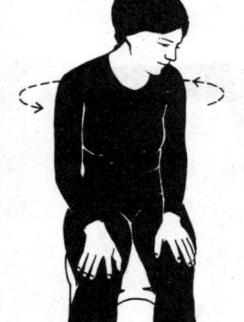

EXERCISE 10.

STARTING POSITION: Sitting.
MOVEMENT: Make a circle in front of the chest with both arms, elbows kept slightly flexed.

EXERCISE 11.

STARTING POSITION: Sitting, hands on knees.
MOVEMENT: Rotate the trunk in a small range.

Exercises for Coronary Heart Disease

EXERCISE 12.

STARTING POSITION: Sitting.
MOVEMENT: Stand up, raise the arms forward and stretch them up to the sides, with palms upward. Then return to the starting position.

EXERCISE 13.

STARTING POSITION: Standing.
MOVEMENT: Step in place for 30 seconds, at a rate of 80–90 steps per minute.

EXERCISE 14.

STARTING POSITION: Standing.
MOVEMENT: 1. Take a step to the left with the left foot and bend the elbows crossed in front of the chest, palms downward. 2. Twist the trunk to the left and stretch the arms out to the sides at shoulder level, elbows straight, palms upward. 3. Bend arms to position 1. 4. Return to the starting position. Repeat the sequence, this time stepping and twisting to the right side.

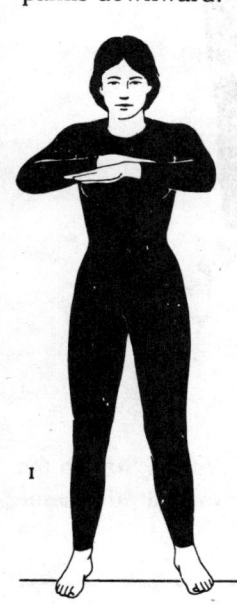

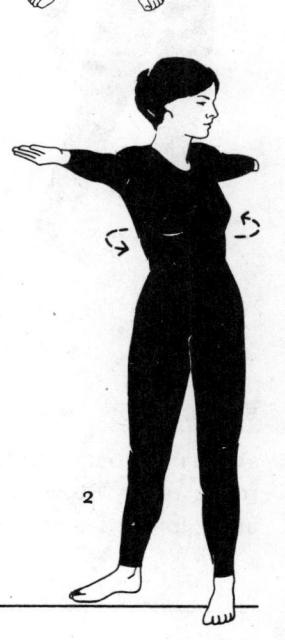

CHINESE THERAPEUTIC EXERCISES

EXERCISE 15.

STARTING POSITION: Standing with feet separated shoulder width.
MOVEMENT: 1. Bend the trunk to the left and bend the right arm up gradually until the right hand, moving along the side, reaches the lower rib region. Then return to the starting position. 2. Bend the trunk to the right and bend the left arm up until the left hand, moving along the side, reaches the lower rib region. And again, return to the starting position.

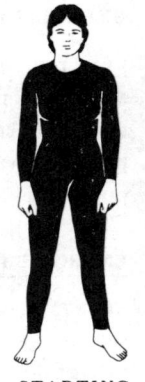

STARTING POSITION

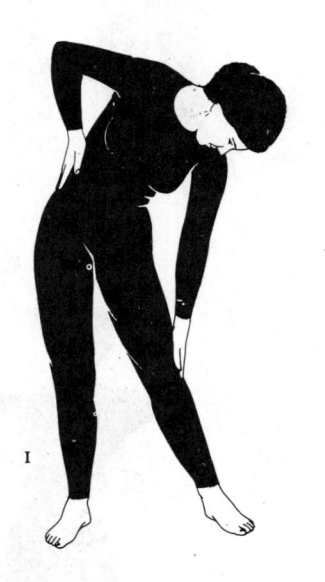

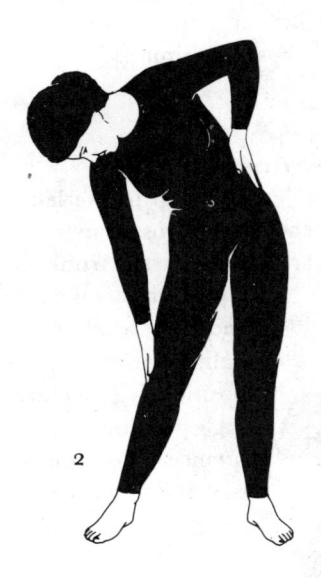

EXERCISE 16.

STARTING POSITION: Standing.
MOVEMENT: "Rowing." 1. Take a step forward with the left foot. Stretch the arms forward and upward, with the trunk falling forward at the same

Exercises for Coronary Heart Disease

time. 2. Then draw the hands downward and backward, with the trunk rising and extending backward at the same time.

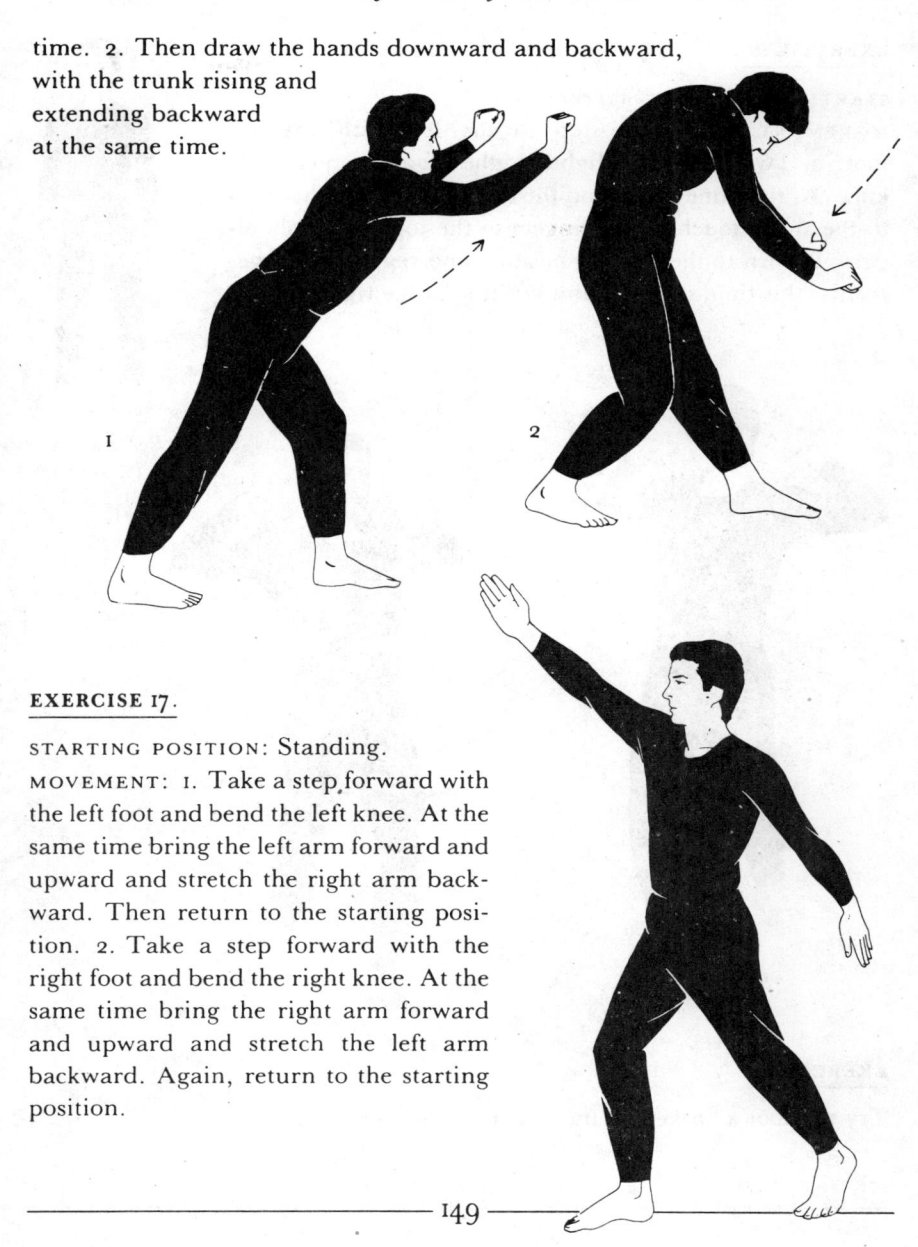

EXERCISE 17.

STARTING POSITION: Standing.

MOVEMENT: 1. Take a step forward with the left foot and bend the left knee. At the same time bring the left arm forward and upward and stretch the right arm backward. Then return to the starting position. 2. Take a step forward with the right foot and bend the right knee. At the same time bring the right arm forward and upward and stretch the left arm backward. Again, return to the starting position.

149

CHINESE THERAPEUTIC EXERCISES

EXERCISE 18.

STARTING POSITION: Standing.
MOVEMENT: 1. Take a step to the left with the left foot. 2. Twist the trunk slightly to the left and bend the left knee. At the same time bend the elbows and raise the arms to the sides, touching the fingers to the tops of the shoulders. Return to the starting position and repeat the movements, this time stepping and twisting to the right side.

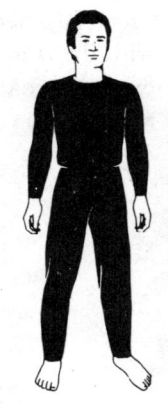

STARTING POSITION

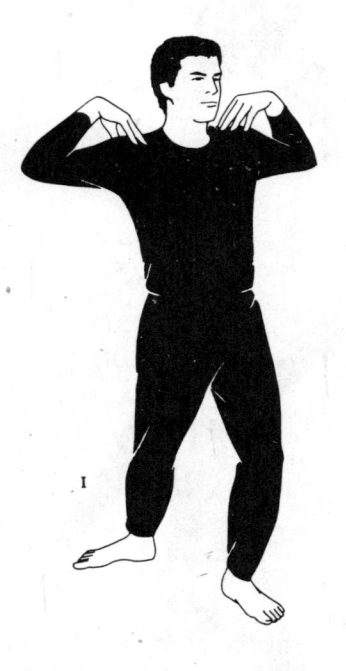

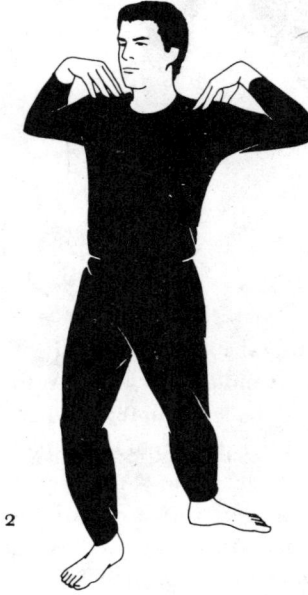

EXERCISE 19.

Try to shoot a basketball into a net, 10–20 shots.

Exercises for Coronary Heart Disease

EXERCISE 20.

Pedal a stationary bicycle without resistance 2–3 minutes.

EXERCISE 21.

STARTING POSITION: Standing.
MOVEMENT: 1. Take a step forward with the left foot and bring the arms upward, palms facing forward, with the trunk slightly extended and the head raised. Then, return to the starting position. 2. Repeat, this time with right foot stepping forward. And again, return to the starting position.

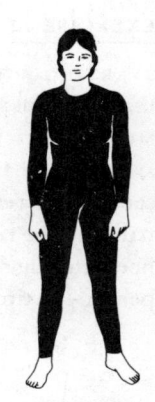

STARTING POSITION

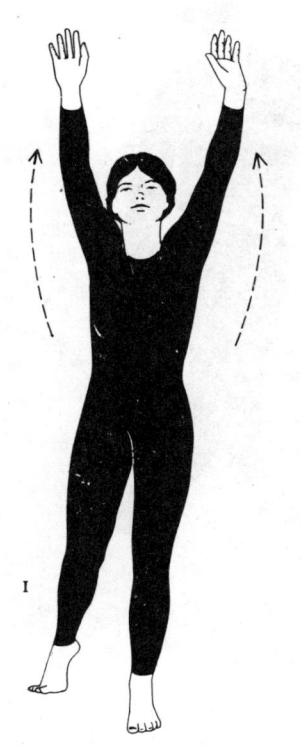

1

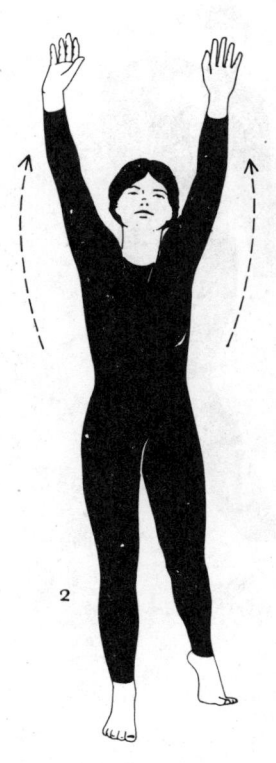

2

CHINESE THERAPEUTIC EXERCISES

EXERCISE 22.

STARTING POSITION: Stride standing (feet separated more than shoulder width), arms bent at the sides, palms down.

MOVEMENT: 1. Twist the trunk to the left, with the arms swinging to the left at the same time until the heels can be seen, then return to the starting position. 2. Now twist the trunk to the right with the arms swinging to the right until the heels can be seen. Again, return to the starting position. Repeat 10-20 times.

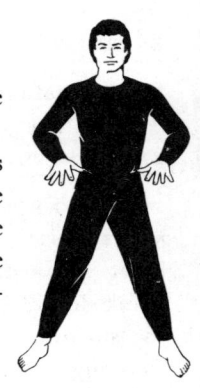

STARTING POSITION

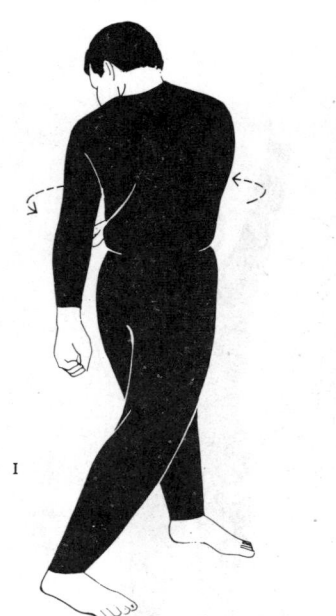

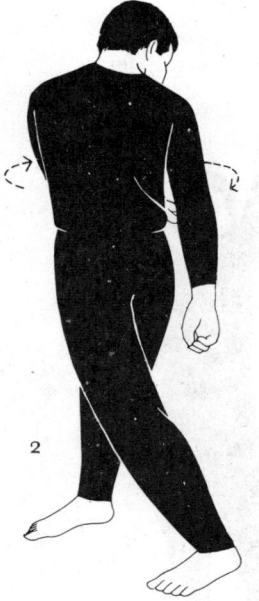

EXERCISE 23.

Walk at a normal rate for 1-1½ minutes.

Exercises for Coronary Heart Disease

EXERCISE 24.

STARTING POSITION: Standing, arms at sides.
MOVEMENT: 1. Raise the arms to the sides, at shoulder level, keeping the elbows straight. At the same time bend and lift the left leg. Then, return to the starting position. 2. Repeat the above, this time bending and lifting the right leg. And again, return to the starting position.

Note: The movements of the arms and legs should be done in a relaxed manner.

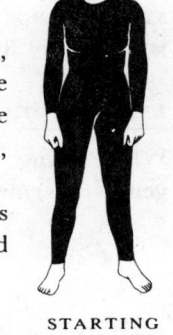

STARTING POSITION

1

2

EXERCISE 25.

STARTING POSITION: Standing.
MOVEMENT: Shrug the shoulders and then relax.

EXERCISE 26.

STARTING POSITION: Standing, keeping hips firm.
MOVEMENT: Breathe slowly and rhythmically for one minute.

EXERCISE 27.

While sitting, massage the head, neck, face, and chest. Use soothing and gentle movements for 3-5 minutes.

Appendix II
A program of therapeutic exercise for patients recovering from acute heart attack

FIRST STAGE (duration: 1-2 weeks): Start with exercises 1 thru 3, then gradually add the other four exercises. In the initial stage, only one session of exercise is scheduled daily. Later, two sessions a day are scheduled. Each of the exercises is to be performed while lying on the back. Repeat each 5-10 times.

EXERCISE 1: Abdominal breathing (gently and easily).

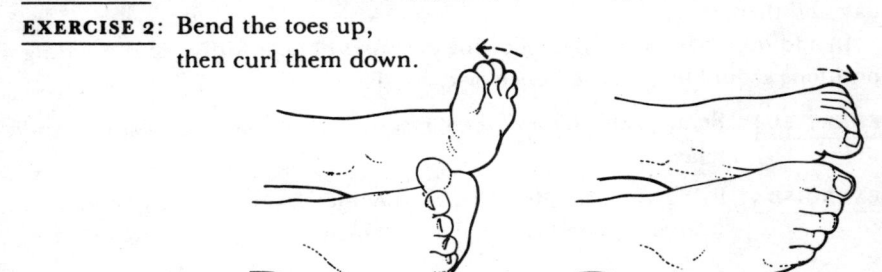

EXERCISE 2: Bend the toes up, then curl them down.

EXERCISE 3: Pull the feet up and then relax; push the feet down and then relax.

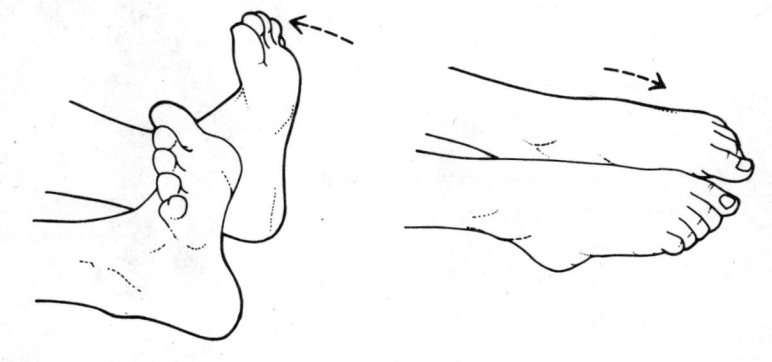

CHINESE THERAPEUTIC EXERCISES

EXERCISE 4: Clench the fists, then relax.
EXERCISE 5: Contract the buttocks, then relax.
EXERCISE 6: Raise the arms above the head, then return them to the starting position.
EXERCISE 7: Bend the legs with the feet sliding on the floor.

SECOND STAGE (duration: 1-2 weeks): During this stage the prescribed exercise is essentially walking. First, walking by the bedside, 5 minutes each session, three times a day. Later, walking in the hospital corridor, 50 yards the first day, 100 yards the second day, 200 the third, and 300 yards the fourth day and thereafter.

In addition to walking, the following exercises done in sitting and standing positions should be practiced once or twice daily.

EXERCISE 1: Bend both elbows, then return to the starting position and relax.
EXERCISE 2: Bring the arms forward to shoulder level keeping the elbows straight. Then bring the arms down.
EXERCISE 3: Make a circle with extended arms and with the elbows bent.

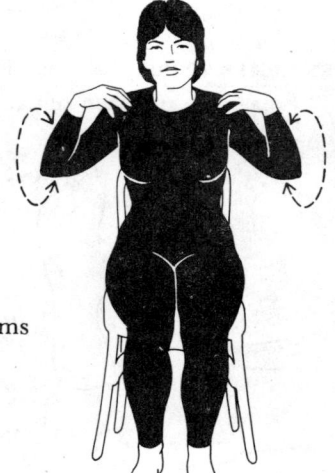

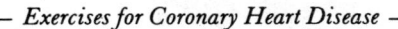

EXERCISE 4: Bend the trunk forward slightly with the arms hanging loosely, then return to the starting position.

EXERCISE 5: Bend the trunk to the left and then to the right, in a small range, while breathing smoothly.

EXERCISE 6: Raise the heels and stand on tiptoe, then return to the starting position with heels resting on the floor.

EXERCISE 7: Raise the legs and step in place.

Finally, the patient may practice stepping up and down stairs, if the physical condition permits. At first, the patient is to step up and down four steps. Then the number of steps is increased in increments of four steps each day or two, up to a maximum of forty steps.

CHAPTER XV

Exercises for Gastrointestinal Problems

Improper life-style involving inactivity and overeating accounts for many gastrointestinal and metabolic diseases. Accordingly, the prevention and treatment of these diseases is largely a matter of improving the undesirable life style. In connection with this, exercise therapy is invaluable. For constipation, indigestion, obesity, and "potbelly"—all symptoms of gastrointestinal problems—a number of therapeutic exercise programs are given in this section.

As *Chi Kung* has been used successfully in China to treat peptic ulcer, it is also included in this section.

Since Chinese exercise therapy has traditionally been much concerned with the prevention of illnesses of the stomach and bowels, two kinds of preventive massage are presented.

However, in the treatment of the above-mentioned disorders, exercise therapy can be successful only when combined with rational dietary regulation.

Chronic constipation

Constipation arising from an irregular life-style, improper diet, and irregular habits of defecation is called chronic constipation. It is commonly seen in those facing a new environment requiring major changes in their life and work habits. However, lack of sufficient physical activity is the most common cause of this type of constipation.

CHINESE THERAPEUTIC EXERCISES

Sedentary working conditions, an irregular life-style, lack of exercise, and ingesting refined, low-fiber foods, all contribute to constipation, because they do not provide adequate stimulus for the bowels to move normally. When these causes are removed, the constipation will be cured.

Exercise therapy is quite effective in treating chronic constipation. Dynamic exercises such as running and jumping can stimulate the movement of the bowels. Abdominal exercise strengthens the abdominal muscles which play an important role in the normal process of defecation. In addition, exercise can alter the neuropsychological state so that neurological regulation of intestinal activity can return to normal.

A variety of therapeutic exercises, therapeutic sports, *Chi Kung,* and massage are indicated for patients with chronic constipation.

Therapeutic exercises

The following exercises which are designed to strengthen the abdominal wall are very helpful:

EXERCISE 1: *Knee bending.*

STARTING POSITION: Lying on the back, arms at sides, palms down. (Whenever lying on the back, a pillow under the head will relax the head and neck, and make breathing easier.)

STARTING POSITION

MOVEMENT: Bend the knees and raise the legs back slowly as close to the chest as possible, then return to the starting position.

Repeat 16 times.

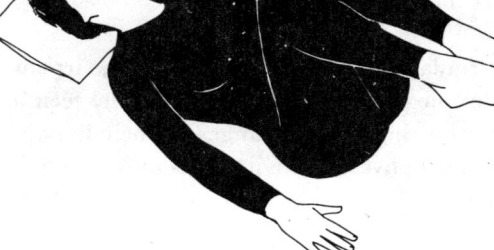

Exercises for Gastrointestinal Problems

EXERCISE 2: *Leg raising*.

STARTING POSITION: Lying on the back, arms at sides with palms down, knees bent close to the chest.

MOVEMENT: Raise legs upward slowly from bent to a vertical position, to where the knees are straight, then return to the starting position. Repeat 16 times.

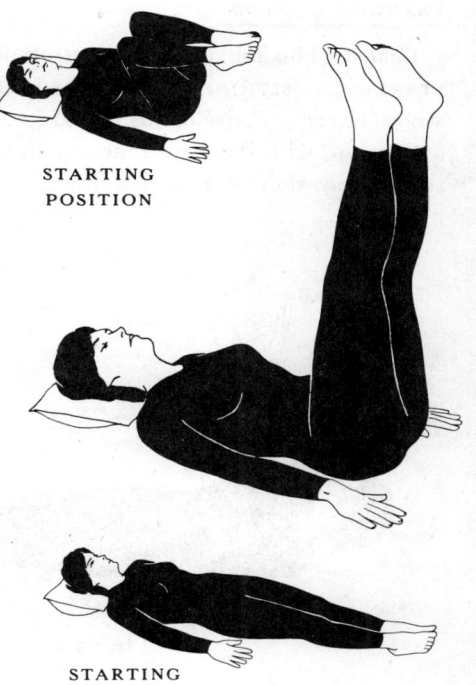

STARTING POSITION

EXERCISE 3: *Cycling*.

STARTING POSITION: Lying on the back, arms at sides, palms down.

STARTING POSITION

MOVEMENT: Bend and stretch out the left and right leg alternately, as in cycling. The exercise should be performed quickly and in as large a range as possible. Keep this up for 20–30 seconds.

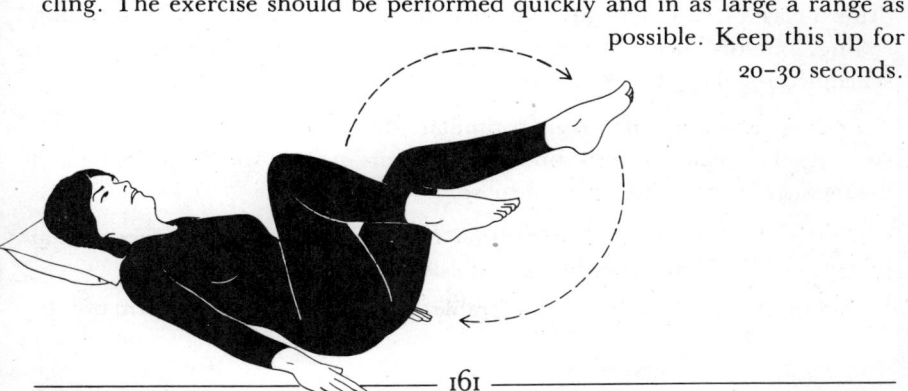

CHINESE THERAPEUTIC EXERCISES

EXERCISE 4: *Sit-ups.*

Caution: This movement is contraindicated for those with back problems.
STARTING POSITION: Lying on the back, palms placed on the floor.
MOVEMENT: 1. Raise hands upward. 2. Then lift head and shoulders slowly and sit up, with the arms reaching forward as far as possible. Return to the starting position. Repeat 6–8 times.

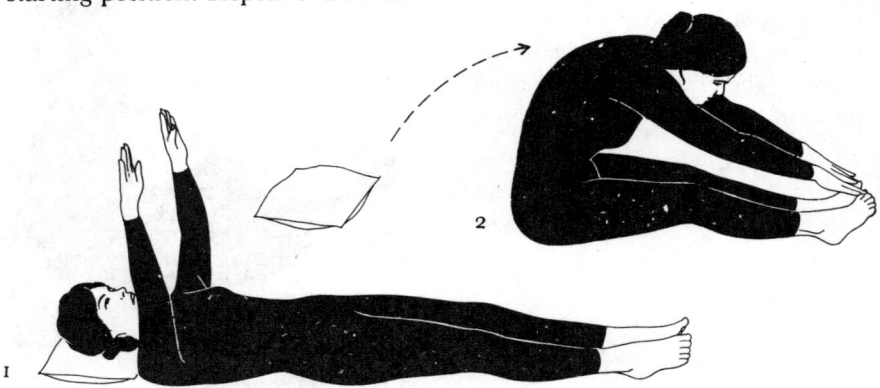

Therapeutic activities

Walking, running, and rowing are preferable.

Walking: Upon rising in the morning, walk briskly for 30 minutes. Then drink a glass of water and go to the toilet to move the bowels. In a sanitorium setting, long-distance walking (approximately 1 mile, or 2 kilometers) may be scheduled regularly for the patient.

Running: Running and jogging stimulate the bowels and promote peristalsis. If level of health permits, one may take part in these sports. Jumping and basketball can serve the same purpose.

Rowing: The movements of rhythmic rowing increase the intra-abdominal pressure, stimulating intestinal peristalsis.

Bathing: A cold water bath is preferable. It may be taken in the form of rubbing the body, a shower, or swimming, depending on the level of fitness and available facilities. If the patient cannot tolerate a cold bath, a hot bath may be taken. However, among these forms of bathing the cold shower is the most effective in stimulating the movement of the bowels. It is recommended that the bath be taken after exercise in the morning.

Chi Kung: For patients with constipation, *Chi Kung for the Internal Organs* is indicated. It should be performed while lying on the back with deep diaphragmatic breathing. This form of *Chi Kung* can "massage" the bowels through intermittent respiration. It has been reported that the range of vertical movement of the diaphragm during *Chi Kung* is 3-4 times greater than during ordinary breathing. This was supported by the finding that under the influence of *Chi Kung* the bowel sounds became louder. In addition, *Chi Kung* may improve the psychological condition, promoting recovery from excessive stress or anxiety, and modifying the bowels' neurological mechanism, return it to normal functioning.

Massage: Self-administered massage on the abdomen is beneficial in cases of chronic constipation. The best position is lying on the back with legs slightly bent, and the knees supported by a pillow. The massage is applied in a circular movement around the umbilicus with the hands on top of each other, starting from the lower right abdomen, moving upward to the upper right abdomen, then across to the lower left abdomen where deep and slow kneading is applied, and finally returning to the lower right abdomen. Repeat this clockwise massage for ten minutes. Upon finishing the massage, stand up, tap the lowest part of the back and the buttocks lightly with both hands. This massage may be applied twice a day after *Chi Kung*.

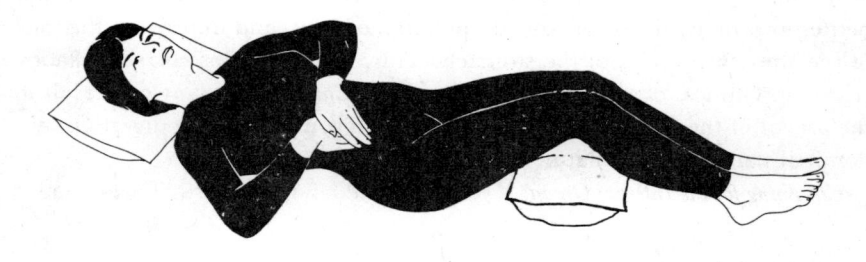

Note: Diet is another aspect in the management of constipation. One should eat foods rich in fiber such as whole grain cereals, fruit, vegetables, whole grain toast or rolls, preserves, and honey, and drink sufficient liquids. No other dietary regulation is necessary.

Gastroptosis

Gastroptosis, the downward displacement of the stomach, will go unnoticed as long as it is symptomless. However, symptoms will occur if the stomach moves down to the lower part of the abdominal cavity, or to the pelvic cavity. The patient usually complains of fullness of the abdomen, indigestion, headache, vertigo, fatigue, and constipation, all resulting from abnormal digestion and absorption, and the ensuing general weakness.

Bodily constitutional factors are said to have a bearing on the development of gastroptosis. It has been found that most patients with gastroptosis are thin and fragile. The ligaments of their abdominal organs are so weak and loose that they cannot keep the stomach in its normal position. Since their abdominal muscles are also very flaccid, the internal organs cannot be prevented from sagging. Other factors leading to gastroptosis are malnutrition, loss of fat tissue in the abdominal cavity, and changes in the shape and volume of the abdominal cavity, found in women after childbirth.

The basic treatment for gastroptosis consists of strengthening the body as well as the abdominal muscles, and improving nutrition. In this regard, *Chi Kung* and therapeutic exercise are very helpful. Therapeutic exercise for gastroptosis emphasizes building up the abdominal muscles (see pages 160–62).

Chi Kung is quite effective in modifying the constitution, increasing the appetite, improving digestion and assimilation of food, and improving the tone of the smooth muscles of the stomach. This, in turn, helps correct a flabby stomach. Clinical observation has shown that *Chi Kung* therapy can result in the ascent of the stomach and relief from such symptoms as indigestion, abdominal pain, fullness, flatulence, and heartburn.

Chi Kung for the Internal Organs is recommended in this regard. The patient is to lie on the back, buttocks supported by a pillow, with the knees bent at an angle between 45–90°. The breathing follows the pattern of diaphragmatic, intermittent respiration (see *Chi Kung for the Internal Organs*, page 74).

Flaccid abdominal wall

A person with a flaccid abdominal wall usually cannot control the bowels, and the abdomen tends to drop forward and downward (sagged abdomen). This sagging belly is often encountered in middle-aged people and in women who have given birth to two or more children.

A sagging belly itself is not a disease. However, it is an underlying factor in many diseases.

Chronic constipation may develop in those with a flaccid abdominal wall, because when evacuating, their abdominal pressure muscles (the external and internal oblique, and rectal muscles) fail to contract forcefully enough to compress the abdomen and stimulate bowel movement.

A great number of people with sagging bellies also complain of lower back pain. This type of functional backache arises from the faulty posture of the back—lordosis. Because of the condition of the belly, the center of their body weight shifts forward. Consequently, the forward curvature of the lumbar spine increases, straining the lower back muscles and causing lower back pain.

Indigestion also is not uncommon in those with a flaccid abdominal wall. It is the result of poor blood circulation in the abdomen as well as weakened peristalsis.

To correct a flaccid abdominal wall, exercise is indispensible. Abdominal exercises are recommended to strengthen the muscles in the abdominal wall. Simple exercises, as those described on pages 160–62, are useful. For those in better physical condition, more vigorous abdominal exercises such as sit-ups with dumbbells or sandbags held in the hands will be more helpful. Deep abdominal (diaphragmatic) breathing is also recommended, with particular emphasis on the strong contraction of the abdominal muscles when breathing out deeply.

CHAPTER XVI

Exercises for Anxiety and Depression

Chinese medicine presumes that physical exercise can have a significant effect on one's state of the mind. Since ancient times exercise has been used in China to foster a tranquil mind and to treat a number of mental disorders, such as depressive states, feelings of sadness, fears (phobias), and anxiety. Traditional Chinese exercise emphasizes training the mind through bodily movement, concentration, and relaxation. Therefore it is also known as "mental exercise" or "spiritual exercise." The traditional Chinese concept of the effect of exercise on the mind is consistent with recent findings by western scientists that exercise may reduce anxiety and depression.

The following section presents exercise programs for patients with anxiety or depression. In these programs, the time-honored Chinese "mental exercises" are incorporated with western remedial games and jogging. These latter activities have recently been reported to be useful in anxiety reduction.

It has been estimated that ten million Americans suffer from anxiety neurosis*, while mental depression is said to be as common as the common cold in the United States.** Various approaches have been tried in coping with these two problems. A century ago, rest therapy was enthusiastically advocated for mental disorders. However, research studies in China and North America over the past twenty years strongly suggest that people with anxiety or depres-

---

* Morgan, W.P., in Proceedings of the National College of Physical Education Association, p. 114, 1973.
** Lawrence, R.M., in Therapeutics Through Exercise (Ed. Lowenthal, D.T. et al), p. 213, 1979.

sion can benefit from exercise training. *Tai Chi Chuan, Chi Kung,* Chinese massage, and western style jogging and remedial games are all recommended for these common emotional disorders.

Tai Chi Chuan

This gentle exercise is particularly effective in training the mind of the exerciser to become quiet, relaxed, and concentrated. Because of this, individuals with anxiety or in low spirits may use it to develop composure and self-confidence. During the practice of *Tai Chi Chuan,* the patient is required to command every movement of the exercise while in deep thought. Irrelevant thoughts, and feelings of anxiety, sadness, and despair will give way to a definite awareness of the concrete benefits of body/mind training. In addition, the gentle and relaxing movements of the exercise can help relieve such physical symptoms as loss of appetite, fullness in the upper abdomen, flatulence, constipation, and vague pains or discomforts in various parts of the body.

Chi Kung

Chi Kung is of benefit to patients with anxiety. Deep and relaxed respiration throughout the practice, in conjunction with mental concentration, brings a sense of relaxation and ease. Furthermore, meditation plays a role akin to psychotherapy during the practice of *Chi Kung.* For example, in order to relieve mental stress and tension, it is recommended in a *Chi Kung* session to recite mentally some words or phrases with a positive connotation and self-suggestive meaning, such as "I am relaxed," "I am getting better day by day," "Worrying is harmful. I might as well take it easy," "I don't have to be so uptight. Everything is going well." On the whole, people with anxiety are recommended to practice *Chi Kung for Fitness* and incorporate the above-mentioned technique of meditation into the practice.

In the experience of Chinese physicians, those with mental depression tend to benefit much more from *Tai Chi* or remedial games than from *Chi Kung.* It seems that a more active and diversified program rather than *Chi Kung* is preferable for these people, as the former produces greater improvement in emotional state and motivation.

Massage

As a symptomatic treatment, massage can bring about a sedative effect. For headaches, massage the face in general and the temporal region in particular. For dizziness or vertigo, tap the occipital region (back of the head) as in "Beating the drum" (page 60). Massage can be self-administered or done by a therapist.

Walking

Clinical observations have shown that for patients with anxiety and depression, long distance walking (approximately 1½ miles, or 2–3 kilometers) can help modify the process of excitation and inhibition in the cerebral cortex. It will also relieve headache and pulsating pain over the temporal region caused by vasomotor dysfunction. Walking is also a refreshing exercise which can raise the spirits of a depressive patient. For older people with heightened tension, a brisk walk attaining a heart rate of about 100 beats per minute, has been shown more effective in reducing neuromuscular tension than was meprobamate, a common tranquilizer.

Jogging and running

Jogging and running are endurance exercises which, with long-term training (more than six weeks), have been shown effective in the treatment of depression and anxiety. In young men and women with moderate depression, running has been found to be just as effective as psychotherapy. A person with mental anxiety who is following a jogging program will become less preoccupied with symptoms and problems. A better subjective feeling, increased self-esteem, and better body image are achieved through participation in a regular jogging program.

The intensity of jogging and running should be adapted to the individual's physical condition. Generally speaking, jogging may be done three times a week, for 30 minutes, and at an acceptable rate—i.e., where the jogger feels relaxed and comfortable. In general, jogging at a rate of about a mile in 20 minutes would be acceptable for emotionally disturbed patients or people with neurotic symptoms.

Remedial games

Patients with depression or anxiety will benefit from stimulating games and sports such as table tennis, basketball, badminton, volley ball, and rowing. Light physical work such as gardening is also helpful.

Caution: 1. In the integrated treatment of anxiety or depression, exercise therapy must be combined with adequate rest, psychotherapy, and medication in order to effect a better cure. In the recovery stage of the illness, exercise alone can be used to keep the patient in a state of positive motivation.

2. Never exercise to the point of exhaustion. Start the exercise program with moderate intensity and increase the effort gradually.

CHAPTER XVII

Exercises for Insomnia

Insomnia has many causes. It is a condition commonly seen in patients with neurosis and transient emotional disturbance. This type of insomnia cannot be treated radically by prescribing a sleeping pill. However, symptomatic treatment of insomnia with exercise is quite simple and effective. What is needed is to calm the overexcited brain cells, leading the cerebral cortex into an inhibitive process, which, in turn, will cause the patient to fall asleep. In this connection, exercise therapy is useful. The following methods have been shown to have sedative effects. They may be regarded as natural "sleeping pills."

Walking

It is well known that walking is the best tranquilizer in the world. It has been reported that insofar as its sedative effect is concerned, 15 minutes of brisk walking is equal to a dosage of meprobamate. For those with insomnia, it is recommended that they walk for 10–15 minutes before going to bed.

Tai Chi Chuan

As a mental exercise, *Tai Chi* can help the patient relax. It is a natural sedative that brings serenity to the mind. Doing a set of *Tai Chi* 30 minutes before going to bed can help overcome insomnia.

Self-administered massage

Sedative self-administered massage is applied when lying in bed ready to go to sleep. The massage used for this condition involves rubbing and stroking the body with both hands by the patient herself or himself. It is also called "the dry bath." First, "wash" (rub) the face lightly with both hands. Next, stroke the left arm with the right hand and the right arm with the left hand. Then stroke the chest and abdomen slowly and lightly. Finally, massage the sole (stroking the point *yung chuan,* see page 64). With this massage, you will very soon become calm. Drowsiness usually occurs in response to a 10-minute session of massage. The next step is to stop the massage, relaxing further into sleep.

Chi Kung

It is recommended to practice *Chi Kung for Relaxation* or *Chi Kung for Fitness* before going to sleep. Lying on the right side is the preferred position. Relax the body, concentrate the mind using the method of "following the breath" (page 72). Practicing *Chi Kung* in this way for 10–15 minutes usually induces drowsiness. *Chi Kung* of this type is called *Chi Kung for Sleep.*

In addition, other adjunctive measures are beneficial, such as immersing the feet in warm water for 20–30 minutes before going to bed as well as stopping reading, writing, or other mental activity 30 minutes before going to bed.

If sleep is still intermittent by midnight, try the method mentioned above once more. It will assist in falling asleep again.

CHAPTER XVIII

Exercises Following Brain Concussion

Brain contusion may occur when the head is severely jarred. In societies with heavy automobile traffic, brain concussion from traffic accidents is not uncommon. Industrial and sports injuries also contribute to the incidence of brain concussion. Exercise therapy is helpful in hastening recovery from these conditions. Sometimes the patient can recover fully with proper rest and other treatment. Quite often, some sequela (after-effects) will remain, such as vertigo, dizziness, headache, absent-mindedness, depression, muscular weakness, or fatigue.

The above-mentioned symptoms may be relieved by exercise therapy in conjunction with medication. Methods of therapeutic exercise used for this condition are much the same as those for anxiety and depression, but with less intensity, because patients recovering from a brain concussion cannot tolerate vigorous exercise. Another valuable treatment is *Chi Kung for Relaxation,* helping to regulate the mental and psychological state of the patient. Walking and doing breathing exercises in the fresh air will make the patient alert and refreshed. Stimulating games such as table tennis and badminton are good for those patients in moderately good physical condition. Exercises accompanied by music can lift the spirits and relieve depression. As a symptomatic treatment, massage on the head performed either by the patient or by a therapist is helpful in relieving headache and vertigo.

CHAPTER XIX

Exercises for Paralysis

This section contains exercises for hemiplegia (paralysis of one side of the body) following stroke, paraplegia (paralysis of the lower half of the body) following spinal cord injury, and palsies resulting from polio.

These programs are not only indicated for patients under medical care in a rehabilitation center, but also for those who have been discharged from a hospital or rehabilitation center and are now at home. A great number of exercises, such as the arm and hand exercises for functional training, and a walking program in the later recovery stage, can also be performed by the patient alone.

It is the experience of Chinese physicians that it is best to combine exercise therapy with acupuncture in the initial stage of rehabilitative treatment (the first six months after the accident causing the paralysis). However, the exercise training should be continued as long as possible, over a period of months or even years.

Massage is a good adjunct to exercise training in the treatment of paralysis. For flaccid muscles, the method of deep kneading or stroking is recommended. For contracted or spastic muscles, soothing surface stroking is indicated.

Exercise therapy in hemiplegia

Cautions: 1. In cases of hemiplegia the intensity of exercise should be very low, so that an extra burden is not put on the cardiovascular system. 2. Pay attention to safety. When doing standing and walking exercises, the patient must be supervised by a therapist or an attendant for support and guidance.

FIRST STAGE: This stage generally begins in the early recovery period, about 3-4 weeks after onset of the attack. The goal during this stage is to restore the functions of sitting and standing. Apart from massage and passive movements applied to the paralytic limbs, the following exercises should be taught to the patient.
- Lying on the back, pull the foot and the toes up as far as possible, then relax.
- Lying on the back with legs extended, flex (bend) the hips and knees, then stretch them to return to the starting position.
- Sitting exercise: Sit up from a lying position, first with the help of a therapist, then gradually on one's own.
- Sitting on a chair, step in place, alternating with the right and left leg.
- Sitting on a chair, stand up from the chair, with hands firmly holding onto a stable object, then sit down.
- Standing exercise: Stand at bedside, with hands firmly holding onto a stable object for balance.
- Standing exercise: Stand alongside the bed, without holding onto any means of support.
- Standing exercise: Stand away from the bed, without relying on any object.

SECOND STAGE: The goal during this stage is to restore the function of walking and to improve the function of the upper extremities, especially the fingers. The ambulation program is as follows:
- Standing, with hands holding onto a stable object, move the trunk to the healthy side, then to the paralytic side. Rest weight alternately on the healthy, then the affected side.

- Standing, with hands holding onto a stable object, step in place.
- Standing, with hands holding onto a stable object, step sideward.
- Walk with the help of a walker.
- Walk with a cane.
- Walk independently.

At this stage, the hand program is as follows:
- Reduce the flexion contracture of the fingers by massage and passive movements.
- Separate the fingers as widely as possible. Try to keep the fingers straight and flat, and touch the surface of a table.
- Separate the fingers from each other, then close them together.
- Exercise the hands and fingers using various kinds of small apparatus.

THIRD STAGE: The goal of this stage is to restore the functions of everyday activity. Further ambulation training includes a variety of complex walking exercises such as walking over obstacles, walking up and down stairs, walking up a slope, and walking at various speeds. The hand program is much the same as that used in the second stage. Those who are recovering faster will do coordination exercises, agility exercises (e.g., grasping and releasing a ball, catching a ball), and other forms of occupational therapy.

Exercise therapy to help paraplegics stand

Paraplegia is the paralysis of the lower half of the body due to disease or injury of the spinal cord. Intensive treatment is important in order to give the paraplegic an opportunity to restore functioning as much as possible and enjoy a longer, more active life.

In the comprehensive treatment of paraplegia, exercise therapy plays a very important role in improving motor function, preventing complications, and maintaining general health.

The following program is applicable to paraplegics in the recovery period, in particular those who have suffered mild spinal injury. In cases of severe spinal injury, surgical intervention is usually indicated, followed by exercise therapy in the postoperative period.

Sitting exercise

The patient is helped to sit up from the supine position. At first, he or she can only assume a half-sitting position with the back leaning against a tilted headrest. This is followed by self-training, with supervision, for maintaining long sitting on the bed (i.e., legs extended flat on a bed or the floor). Finally, the patient is taught to sit on the side of the bed with both feet hanging over the edge. Sometimes the patient will experience a sense of syncope (faintness) when sitting up straight, particularly during several of the earlier sessions. This is due to ischemia (deficient blood supply) in the brain as a result of poor vasomotor response. It may be overcome by preparatory training, in the form of turning the body around and changing position frequently while lying in bed. When doing the sitting exercise, it is recommended that a belt be fastened to the abdomen to prevent a sudden influx of blood into the abdomen from the brain.

Preparation for getting off the bed

Before transferring from the bed to a chair or wheelchair, the patient is taught to do conditioning exercises to strengthen the muscles of the back, arms, and shoulder girdle. A kneeling exercise is also very important to train the knees to bear weight.
- Lying on the stomach, raise the body to an elbow-knee position, and crawl forward on the bed by moving the hip joint.
- Elbow-knee position ("four point" kneeling). Supported by two cut-down crutches (half the length of regular crutches), raise the body to assume a kneel-standing position. Then move the hip joints forward and backward to prepare for walking on the knees.

Standing exercise

The following procedures are training for standing.
- Prone standing, the trunk leaning on a bed, with the chest supported by pillows.
- Standing on a tilt table for 30 minutes at an angle of 45-70°.
- Standing with crutches, the back leaning against a wall and the knees supported by the hands of a therapist.
- As above, but without the support of a therapist.
- Standing between parallel bars with hands firmly holding the bars.
- Standing with the support of crutches.
- Standing with the support of a therapist.
- Standing independently.

Walking exercise

When the patient can stand with crutches or with the support of a therapist, he or she may be taught to walk according to the following program:
- Walking between parallel bars or with a walker, the hands holding firmly onto the bar.
- Walking with crutches, the knees supported by a therapist or by a brace.
- Walking with crutches.
- Walking with two canes.
- Walking with one cane.
- Walking independently.

For other exercises used in training patients to stand and walk, see *Exercise therapy in hemiplegia: third stage* (page 177).

The patient must be given help and supervision during both the standing sessions and walking exercises to prevent falling.

In spite of the fact that most paraplegics can benefit to varying degrees from exercise therapy, a great number still have to rely on the support of crutches or braces. Consequently, they must be taught to walk properly with crutches. There are two basic types of crutch gait for paraplegics:

1. The "four-pointed" gait. When walking with this type of gait, one crutch is advanced, then the opposite foot, then the other crutch, and then the other foot. This is a very stable gait, moving slowly, always leaving three points on the floor at one time. However, for patients with high spastic lesions, this type of gait is extremely difficult to perform.

2. The "shuffle-to and swing-to" gait: This consists of advancing both crutches forward at the same time and then dragging the feet toward the crutches. The feet are always behind the crutches.

The preceding principles and methods of exercise therapy are also applicable to paraplegics recovering from transverse myelitis.

Therapeutic sports

In recent years an increasing number of paraplegic patients in wheelchairs have taken part in various sports, not only at continuing care centers or at the spinal centers, but also at the international athletic meets especially organized for the handicapped.

Indeed, paraplegics are capable of playing a variety of games and sports. Participation in some sports is actually a necessity to the paraplegic's life and health. Since they have lost the ability to run, jump, and walk, they have lost the opportunity to participate in many of the physical activities which healthy people enjoy daily. If they do not exercise their remaining healthy limbs, their general health as well as their arm and trunk muscles will be weakened. Therapeutic sports can develop muscle tone, increase the strength of the muscles in the arms, back, and abdomen, and improve the general physical condition. The well developed arms and shoulder girdle are valuable assets to paraplegics, which will help them overcome many inconveniences encountered in their daily wheelchair life. Anyone who watches paraplegics in wheelchairs playing therapeutic sports in high spirits and with impressive vitality will realize that they can and should take part in physical training.

Many games involving the use of the arms and trunk are of value to paraplegics. For example, dumbbell exercises, ball-throwing, table-tennis, archery, and basketball-shooting are good for building up the muscles in the shoulder girdle and back. Among these, archery is particularly valuable, because of its effect of strengthening the muscles in the trunk and upper arms that are very important for daily activities. As well, archery can help correct scoliosis (when the thoracic curve is on the right side, the right hand should be used to draw the bow) and can improve sitting balance.

Therapeutic sports may be done individually, at home, or in a group setting at a rehabilitation center.

Exercise therapy in poliomyelitis

Polio (acute anterior poliomyelitis), commonly known as infantile paralysis, is the inflammation of the gray matter of the spinal cord. Since the disease destroys the cells that send messages from the brain to the muscles (the anterior horn cells), the affected muscles are denervated (without nerve supply) and become paralytic. The muscles in the lower limbs are most frequently involved. The patient, usually a child, cannot walk properly, with atrophy of the muscles, and contracture and deformity of the limb. In an exercise program for the treatment of this condition, the re-education of the paralytic muscles through specific exercises, in conjunction with massage, is emphasized. Focus is placed on the quadriceps, anterior tibial muscle, iliopsoas, peroneal, and gluteal muscles, which are frequently affected and lose their normal functioning to varying degrees.

Exercises for building up the quadriceps

The primary function of the quadriceps is to extend the knee. Persons with paralytic quadriceps are unable to extend the affected knee or to keep it straight to bear the body weight when standing and walking. Normal walking is impossible for many post-polio patients, since the paralytic quadriceps cannot sustain the body weight. Usually, hyper-extended deformity of the knee will develop (i.e., the knee will bend backward when standing, and tends to snap backward suddenly with each step).

The exercise program for building up the quadriceps is as follows:

- Sitting on the floor or on a chair, with the knee straight, contract the quadriceps as hard as possible to pull the knee cap up, and then relax with the knee cap back in the original position. When contracting the knee, the foot remains on the floor. The patient should practice ten-second contractions for five minutes each hour while awake.
- While sitting with the knee bent at a right angle, extend the leg as far as possible with the assistance of the hands.
- While sitting with the knee bent, extend the leg so as to kick a ball placed in front of the foot.
- While sitting with the knee kept straight, the straight leg is raised as far as possible and then slowly lowered. As the patient becomes stronger, weight is added by means of a weight-bag draped over the ankle.

Exercises for building up the anterior tibial muscle

The primary function of the anterior tibial muscle is to dorsiflex (bend upward) the foot. Drop-foot usually develops after the muscle has been paralyzed. The exercise program for strengthening this muscle is as follows:

- While sitting, pull the foot up in dorsiflexion as hard as possible, using the hand to assist.
- Repeat the above, but without assistance.
- While standing, with the hands holding onto a stable object for support, raise the front of the foot. The heel must be kept flat on the floor.
- Walk, stepping on the heels only.

Exercises for strengthening the peroneal muscle

The primary function of the peroneal muscle is eversion of the foot (turning the foot outward). If this muscle is paralyzed, the foot cannot evert, and pes varus (the deformity of the inversion of the foot) will develop. The following exercises are designed to strengthen the muscle and to correct inversion of the foot.

- While sitting, raise the lateral edge of the foot as forcefully as possible, while the medial (inner) edge of the foot remains touching the floor.
- While sitting, with legs close together, try to turn the foot outward so as to separate the feet as much as possible. While doing this, the knees remain close to each other, and the medial edges of the feet remain touching the floor.

Exercises for strengthening the ilio-psoas

The primary function of the ilio-psoas is to flex the hip. If this muscle is paralyzed, the hip cannot be flexed upward. The patient is advised to do the following re-education exercises:

1. While lying on the side, flex the thigh, moving the hip towards the abdomen.

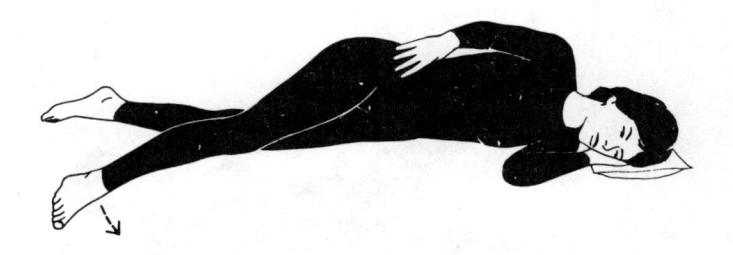

2. While lying on the back, flex the hip and knee. The heel remains touching the floor.

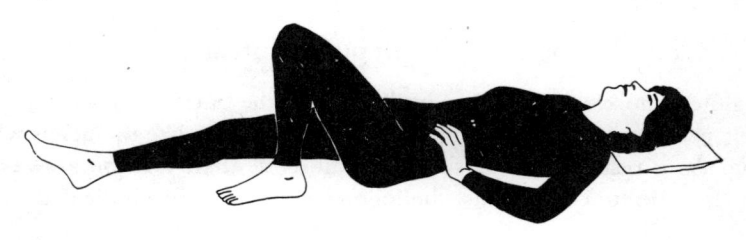

— CHINESE THERAPEUTIC EXERCISES —

3. While lying on the back, flex the hip and knee, bringing the thigh towards the chest. The foot is raised up from the floor.

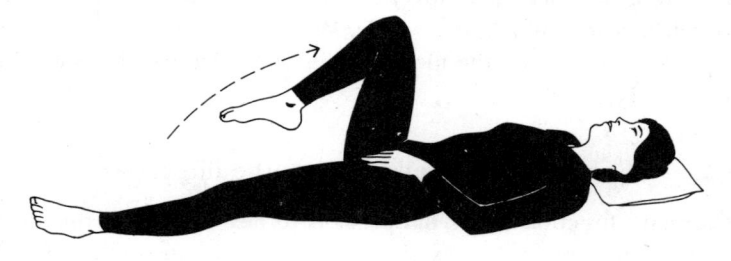

4. While lying on the back, raise the leg up with the knee kept as straight as possible.

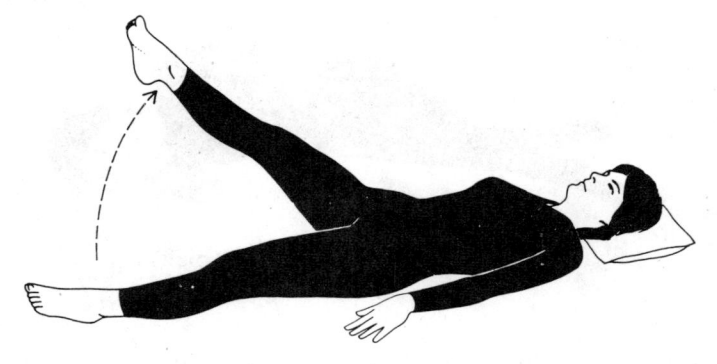

Exercises for strengthening the gluteal muscles

The gluteal muscles are located in the area of the buttocks and hip joints, and their primary function is to extend the hip and stabilize the pelvis when standing. As a result of paralysis of the muscles, there will be a swaying posture. In order to correct this, the following exercises are indicated:

Exercises for Paralysis

1. While lying on the back, tighten the glutei, pulling the buttocks toward the center of the body.
2. While lying on the stomach, raise each leg, keeping the knee straight.

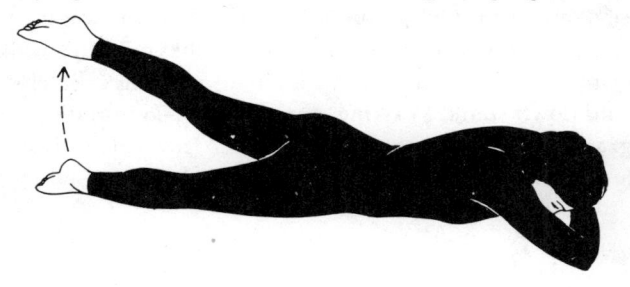

3. While lying on the back, extend the leg out to the side, keeping the knee straight.

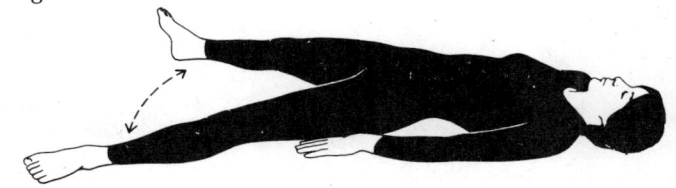

In addition to the preceding exercises which are specifically for the paralytic muscles, combined movements involving different groups of muscles should be performed to develop efficiency in daily activities.

General calisthenics: These exercises should include arm and shoulder girdle movements in the sitting position, back muscle exercises in the prone (face downward) lying position, abdominal muscle exercises in the supine (on the back) lying position, and crawling exercises in the quadruped position.

Weight-bearing exercises: The purpose of weight-bearing exercises is to develop stability in standing and walking. The patient is asked to shift position from sitting on the heels to kneeling. Later, he or she is asked to stand up from a squatting position.

Play activities: Pedaling a tricycle, kicking a ball with the knees while kneeling.

Walking: At first, the patient, usually a child, learns to walk normally with the assistance of a therapist who supports the child by holding the hands and forearms. Later, the child learns to walk with crutches or with a walker, gradually progressing to walking around in a circle, walking over obstacles and walking up and down stairs. Walking sessions last 5–10 minutes in the initial stage, and gradually increase to 20–30 minutes. Intervals of rest should be scheduled during the session to avoid fatigue.

CHAPTER XX

Exercises for Sciatica and Lumbar Disk Problems

Sciatica is a condition characterized by pain, tingling, and other abnormal sensations in the hip, thigh, leg, and foot, caused by impairment of the sciatic nerve. A variety of conditions are responsible for this. Of these, inflammation of the sciatic nerve, intervertebral disk problems, and lumbosacral arthritis are among the most common.

Inflammation of the sciatic nerve (sciatic neuritis) is commonly caused by exposure to cold, toxicity and infection of the adjacent tissues, and sacroiliac arthritis. When the acute symptoms of sciatic neuritis have lessened, the patient may start massage and therapeutic exercise. The following program offers therapeutic exercises for sciatica of this type.

The treatment is also useful in recovery (post-operative or non-operative) from lower back and leg pain due to lumbar disk problems.

Massage

Tap the lower back, buttocks, and the posterior aspect of the thigh with one end of a stick which is fitted with rubber or cloth for 5–10 minutes, 3–5 times daily. This is generally self-administered by the patient, in a standing position. It may also be performed by a therapist.

Therapeutic exercise

During the initial recovery period, do the following four exercises.

EXERCISE 1: While lying on the back, with legs bent at the knees, open and close the knees. Resistance may be applied on the lateral sides of the knees.

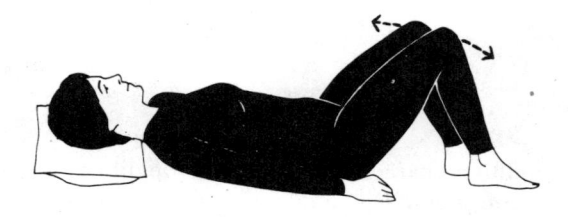

EXERCISE 2: While lying on the back, with legs bent at knees, stretch the legs alternately (heels remain touching the floor).

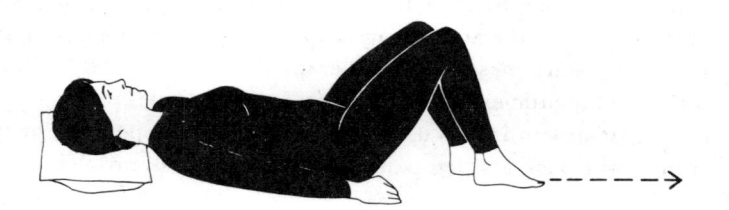

EXERCISE 3: While lying on the healthy side, flex the knee and extend the affected leg. The hip is kept slightly flexed.

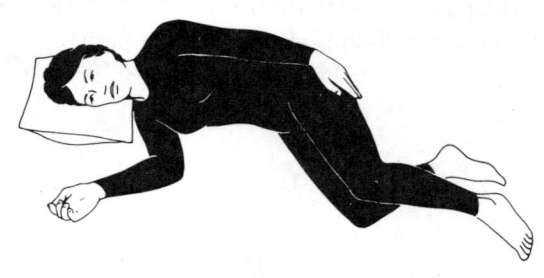

Exercises for Sciatica and Lumbar Disk Problems

EXERCISE 4: While half raised, supporting the body with the hands on the bed behind the body, 1. flex the left knee, extending the leg, 2. then do the same with the right knee and leg.

When the condition has improved, the following exercises may be added:

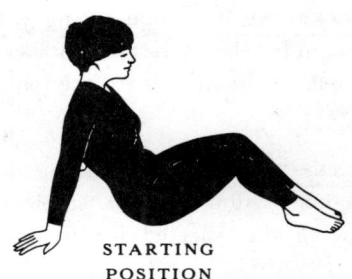

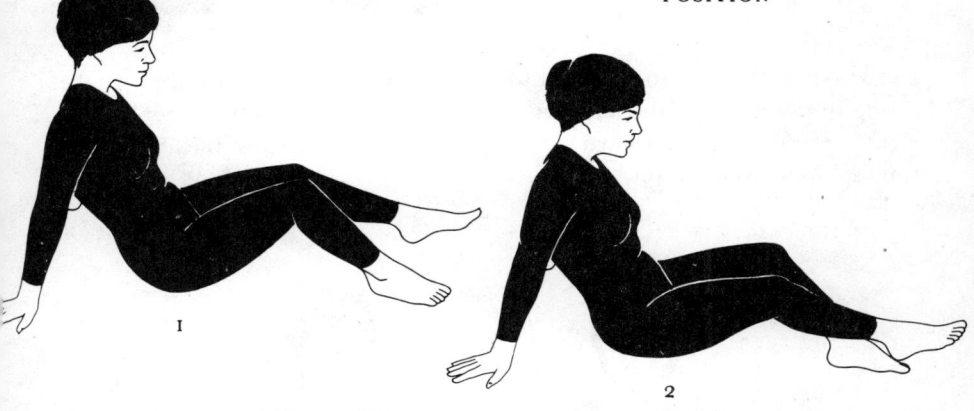

STARTING POSITION

1

2

EXERCISE 5: While sitting on a chair, with knees and hips bent at a right angle and hands on the thighs, bend the trunk forward and slide the hands down the front of the legs simultaneously.

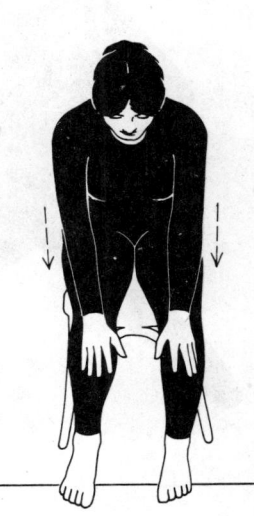

CHINESE THERAPEUTIC EXERCISES

EXERCISE 6: While sitting with legs extended, bend the trunk forward and push the hands toward the toes.

EXERCISE 7: While standing with one hand holding onto a stable object, swing the affected leg forward and backward.

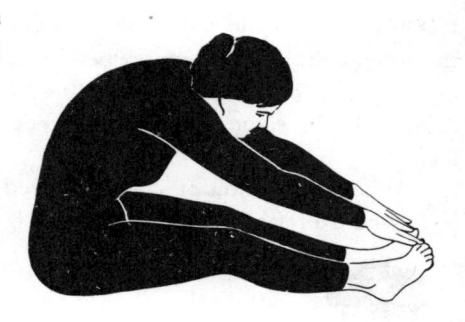

EXERCISE 8: While standing, feet together, hands on hips, hips firm, 1. take a step to the left with the left foot. 2. Next, bend the left knee, keeping the right leg straight. Then return to the starting position. Repeat the above, this time stepping to the right.

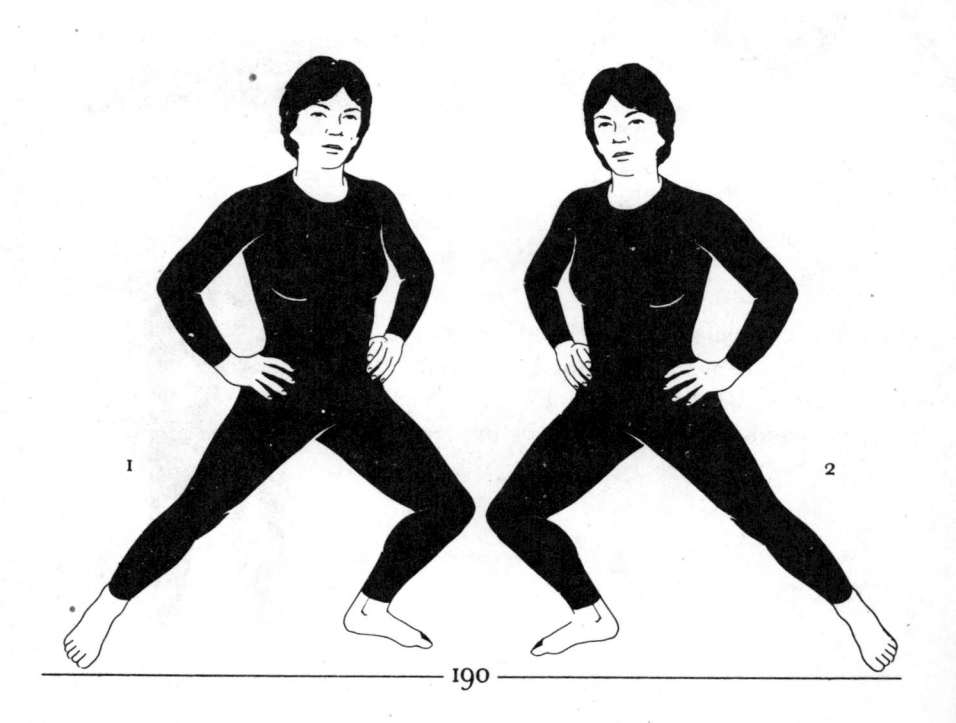

Exercises for Sciatica and Lumbar Disk Problems

EXERCISE 9: While standing, feet apart about shoulder width, hands on hips, hips firm, bend the trunk forward gradually with the knees kept straight.

Sciatica that is due to disk problems (disk degeneration or protrusion) can sometimes be relieved by proper rest followed by therapeutic exercise.

If the protrusion of the nucleus in the intervertebral disk is slight, bed rest for a few days (occasionally more than ten days) will help the protruded nucleus return to its normal position. The sciatica will then disappear. At such time, stretching exercise in a standing position is of help. The trunk is never to be bent forward with the legs straight. Physiotherapy, in the form of a hot pad or infrared radiation, will relieve tension in the back muscles and its attendant pain.

If the protrusion of the nucleus is severe, manipulation and simple stretching exercises may be tried in addition to bed rest. Chiropractic manipulation should be performed by an experienced and skillful professional. One of the simple stretching exercises used in traditional Chinese medicine is "Hanging and swinging" which is done with a wall bar. Standing with feet together, the patient raises the hands upward as far as possible and grasps the bar overhead in order to straighten the trunk. Elbows and legs are also kept straight. The patient then twists the waist 10 times in a clockwise circular movement, then 10 times in a counterclockwise circular movement. This is to be repeated 2-3 times daily. This stretching exercise may help the nucleus return to its normal position. If the pain is not relieved after 10 days of bed rest, stretching exercise, and chiropractic manipulation, these treatments should be discontinued, and the patient advised to consult an orthopedic surgeon for surgical intervention, or other forms of therapy.

INDEX

A

Abdomen
  flaccid abdominal wall, 165
  massage, 63, 102, 163
  relief from pain in, 63, 164, 168
  strengthening and developing, 115, 160-62, 164, 165, 185
Abdominal breathing. *See* Breathing: abdominal
ABDOMINAL BREATHING, 106
Absent-mindedness, relief from, 173. *See also* Mental concentration
Acupressure. *See* Acupuncture points, massage of
Acupuncture for paralysis, 175
Acupuncture points, massage of
  chu san li, 103
  dan tian, 63
  feng chi, 60
  shen shu, 63, 103
  yung ch'uan, 64, 104, 129, 172
Agility, developing, 85, 177. *See also* Flexibility; Strengthening and developing
Anger, relief from, 54. *See also* Emotional state; Relaxation
Angina pectoris, 121, 135, 136, 139
Ankles
  flexibility, 95
  strengthening and developing, 88, 118
Anterior tibial muscle, strengthening, 132
Anxiety and depression, 167-70. *See also* Emotional state; Mental concentration; Relaxation; Wellbeing, promoting
  exercises for, 167-70
    Chi Kung, 168-69
    Tai Chi Chuan, 168
  games for, 167, 168, 169-70
  massage for, 168, 169
  mental and physical relaxation, 167-68
  relief from, 54, 66, 139, 167, 173
Appetite, restoring, 168
Apprehension, relief from, 54. *See also* Emotional state; Mental concentration; Relaxation
Arms
  massage, 117
  strengthening and developing, 39, 41, 44, 45, 49, 53, 57, 84, 92, 101, 114, 178, 185
Arteriosclerosis, 131-34. *See also* Circulation; Coronary heart disease
  defined, 131
  diabetes and, 131

193

INDEX

emotional state and, 131
exercises for, 131–33
　benefits, 131–32
　Tai Chi Chuan, 132
massage for, 134
physical activity and, 131
prevention, 131
Arthritis, 20, 61, 187
Atherosclerosis, 20, 131, 137. *See also* Arteriosclerosis
Athletes. *See also* Flexibility; Strengthening and developing
exercises for, 112–17
　benefits, 9, 11, 111
　Forward thrust, 114
　Hanging and swinging, 116
　Relaxing the waist and tapping the body, 116-17
　Riding a horse, 112
　Swallow flying, 115
　Tiger walking, 113
　Wall pushing, 115
massage for, 111, 117–18
Autogenic healing. *See* Mental concentration; Relaxation; Visualization
Autonomic nervous system. *See* Nervous system

B

Back. *See also* Backache; Posture; Spine
injuries, 86, 113
massage, 163
pain, 165
　prevention of, 11, 93, 114, 116
　relief from, 187–91
problems, 56, 62, 92, 162, 165
strengthening and developing, 41, 53, 62, 87, 111, 115, 178, 180, 185
Backache. *See also* Back; Posture; Spine
as side effect of *Chi Kung*, 68
prevention, 56, 97, 98, 99, 100, 103, 115

treatment, 63, 106
Ba Duan Jin (Eight fine exercises), 9, 11, 13, 49–58
benefits of, 11, 49
for the chronically ill, 49
for the elderly, 49
exercises, 51–58
　Curing the five troubles and seven disorders by turning the head backward and gazing sternly, 54
　Increasing the vital energy by tightening the fists and gazing sternly, 57
　Keeping all diseases away by raising the heels seven times, 58
　Regulating the internal organs by raising both hands to the sky, 50
　Regulating the spleen and stomach by raising the hand upward, 53
　Shooting the eagle by drawing the bow with the hands, 51–52
　Strengthening the loins and kidneys by bending forward with hands touching the feet, 56
　Tranquilizing the fiery heart by turning the head around and swinging the hips, 55
how to practice, 49
Balance, improving, 21, 123, 124, 181
Bathing, 162
BEATING THE "DRUM OF HEAVEN," 60
BENDING FORWARD, 47
BENDING THE TRUNK WITH THE HANDS TOUCHING THE FEET, 62
BITING THE TEETH, 60
Blood. *See* Arteriosclerosis; Circulation; Coronary heart disease; Hypertension
Blood pressure, high. *See* Hypertension
Bowel illness, prevention of, 159, 163. *See also* Gastrointestinal problems
BOWING, 46

INDEX

Brain concussion, exercises following, 173
Breathing
 abdominal, 21, 41, 72-73, 106, 155, 165
 in Chi Kung, 65, 66-67, 68, 69-70, 72, 73, 74, 75
 in anxiety and depression, 168
 in brain concussion, 173
 in coronary heart disease, 155
 counting the breaths, 72
 following the breath, 72
 diaphragmatic. *See* Breathing: abdominal
 difficulty, 68
 exercise, traditional Chinese, 78
 improving, 20, 36, 50, 75, 78, 94, 165
 in gastrointestinal problems, 163, 165
 in hypertension, 78, 122, 123, 125, 128
 in insomnia, 172
 in pregnancy, 108
 in *Tai Chi Chuan,* 20, 21, 165
 in *Yi Jin Jing,* 36
Buttocks, strengthening and developing, 184-85

C

Calcific arteriosclerosis, 131. *See also* Arteriosclerosis
Calisthenics, 35, 49, 78, 185
Calves, strengthening and developing, 58, 87
Cardiorespiratory fitness, 83, 94. *See also* Breathing; Heart; Lungs
Chest
 massage, 154
 pain, 68, 121, 135, 136, 139, 164
 strengthening and developing, 36, 37, 38, 49, 51, 61, 62, 94
Chi Kung (Invigorating exercises), 7, 65-75. *See also Chi Kung for Fitness; Chi Kung for the Internal Organs;*

Chi Kung for Relaxation; Chi Kung for Sleep; Standing Chi Kung
 for anxiety and depression, 168-69
 benefits of, 11, 65-67
 breathing in, 65, 66-67, 68, 69, 72
 for constipation, 160
 for coronary heart disease, 135, 139
 defined, 65
 as "energy-saving" exercise, 65
 for gastrointestinal problems, 159-64, 165
 how to practice, 66-67
 for hypertension, 121, 122-24
 for insomnia, 172
 longevity and, 65
 meditation in, 65
 mental concentration in, 65, 66, 67, 69, 70, 72
 for mental and physical relaxation, 65, 66
 for peptic ulcer, 159
 possible side effects, 67-69
 principles of, 65-67
Chi Kung for Fitness, 12, 65, 70-73, 172
 benefits of, 70
 breathing in, 70, 72-73
 exercises, 71
 frequency and length of training, 73
 for hypertension, 70, 122
 principles of, 70
 program for the practice of, 73
 for psychoneuroses, 70
 quietness training, 73
Chi Kung for the Internal Organs, 65, 74-75
 benefits of, 74
 breathing in, 74-75
 for constipation, 74, 163
 for gastroptosis, 74, 164
 for peptic ulcer, 74
 principles of, 74-75
 quietness training, 75
 for viral hepatitis, 74

INDEX

Chi Kung for Relaxation, 13, 65, 69-70, 172
  for brain concussion, 173
  breathing in, 69
  benefits of, 69
  in chronic illness, 69
  frequency and length of training, 70
  for hypertension, 122
  principles of, 69-70
  quietness training, 69-70, 122
Chi Kung for Sleep, 172
Children
  exercises for, 83-88
    benefits, 8, 11, 83
    Edge walking, 88
    Eye massage, 88
    Hitting the bean bag, 84
    Monkey play, 85
    Rope jumping, 84
    Tiger walking, 86
    Tip-toe walking, 87
    Worm wriggling, 87
Chilliness, relief from, 54
Chinese exercise therapy, 7-10. *See also* Chinese fitness exercises; Chinese therapeutic exercise; Traditional Chinese exercises
  as body/mind technique, 8
  massage and, 8
  medical principles, 8
  mental concentration and, 8
  physiological principles, 8
  psychological principles, 8
  as preventive care, 9
  symbolic implications, 8
Chinese fitness exercises, 81-118
  benefits of, 7-13
  for athletes, 111-18
  for children, 83-88
  for the elderly, 97-104
  for pregnant women, 105-10
  for the sedentary, 89-95

Chinese therapeutic exercises, 119-91
  benefits of, 7-13
  for anxiety and depression, 167-70
  for arteriosclerosis, 131-34
  following brain concussion, 173
  for coronary heart disease, 135-57
  for gastrointestinal problems, 159-65
  for hypertension, 121-29
  for insomnia, 171-72
  for paralysis, 175-81
  for sciatica and lumbar disk problems, 187-91
Chronic constipation. *See* Constipation
Chronic illness, 8, 9, 12, 49, 59, 69, 78, 79
Chu san li acupoint, 103
CIRCLING AT A RESTING POSITION, 79
CIRCLING WHILE MOVING THE LEGS UP AND DOWN, 79
CIRCLING WHILE WALKING, 80
Circulation. *See also* Arteriosclerosis; Coronary heart disease; Heart
  in abdomen, *Tai Chi Chuan* and, 20
  fibrinolysis, 137
  flaccid abdominal wall and, 165
  improving, 9, 11, 20, 60, 64, 90, 95, 98, 101, 102, 109, 131-32, 136-37
  ischemia, 132, 136, 178
  in paraplegia, 178
Concentration. *See* Mental concentration
Constipation
  causes of, 159-60
  diet for, 164
  exercises for, 159, 160-62
    Chi Kung for the Internal Organs, 74, 163
  flaccid abdominal wall, 165
  massage for, 163
  relief from, 164, 168
  therapeutic activities, 162-63
  treatment, 159

INDEX

Coordination, improving, 21, 85, 124, 177
Coronary artery disease. *See* Coronary heart disease
Coronary heart disease, 7, 135-57. *See also* Arteriosclerosis; Circulation
  age and, 136
  angina and, 135, 136, 139
  blood pressure and, 139
  circulation and, 135, 136, 137, 138
  defined, 136
  diet and, 135, 136
  emotional state and, 139
  exercises for, 11, 135-57
    benefits, 137-38
    Chi Kung, 135, 139
    precautions, 135
    preventive exercises, 135-38
    Tai Chi Chuan, 135, 139
    therapeutic exercise, 139-40, 141-54, 155-57
  games for, 139
  heart attack, 135, 136-37, 140
    exercise program for recovering patients, 155-57
  massage for, 154
  mental and physical relaxation, 135, 137
  and metabolism, 137
  and the sedentary, 89
  symptoms, 135-37
COW LOOKING AT THE MOON, THE, 99
CURING THE FIVE TROUBLES AND SEVEN DISORDERS BY TURNING THE HEAD BACKWARD AND GAZING STERNLY, 54
CYCLING, 161

D

Dan tian acupoint, 63
Depression. *See* Anxiety and depression
Diaphragm, strengthening, 50, 53, 163. *See also* Breathing
Diaphragmatic breathing. *See* Breathing: abdominal
Diet
  and coronary heart disease, 135, 136
  and gastrointestinal problems, 159, 160, 164
  importance of, 136, 159
Digestion, improving, 20, 53, 90, 92, 98, 102, 109, 164. *See also* Gastrointestinal problems
Disk problems. *See also* Back; Backache; Posture; Spine
  chiropractic manipulation for, 191
  exercises for, 187-91
  physiotherapy, 191
  surgical intervention, 191
Dizziness. *See also* Vertigo
  prevention, 46
  relief from, 20, 54, 60, 121, 129, 139, 169, 173
DRAGON STAMPING ON THE EARTH, THE, 100
DRAWING A BOW, 62
Drowsiness, as side effect of *Chi Kung*, 68
"Dry bath," 172
Dyspepsia, relief from, 132

E

Edema, relief from, 110
EDGE WALKING, 88
Elderly, the
  Ba Duan Jin and, 49
  coronary heart disease and, 136
  exercises for, 97-104
    benefits, 8, 9, 11, 13, 97
    The cow looking at the moon, 99
    The dragon stamping on the earth, 100
    Half-squatting, 101

INDEX

Handling two chestnuts with one hand, 101
Rowing, 100
Swinging the arms, 98
Walking and massaging the abdomen, 102
massage for, 102-4
Shier Duan Jin and, 59
Electrocardiogram, 136
Emotional state, 7-9, 19, 55, 69, 121, 137, 168-69. *See also* Anxiety and depression; Mental concentration; Relaxation
arteriosclerosis and, 131
coronary heart disease and, 139
gastrointestinal problems and, 163
insomnia and, 171
Emphysema, 70. *See also* Lungs
Exercises. *See* Calisthenics; Chinese fitness exercises; Chinese therapeutic exercises; Flexibility; Games and sports, therapeutic; Hiking and hill climbing; Jogging; Rowing; Strengthening and developing; Swimming; Terrain cure; Traditional Chinese exercises; Walking; specific ailments and individual parts of the body.
Extreme climate, relief from, 54
Eyesight, improving, 88

F

Face massage, 60, 129, 154
Faintness, 178
as side effect of *Chi Kung*, 69
Fatigue, relief from, 21, 164, 173. *See also Chi Kung*
Feet
massage, 64, 104, 129
numbness, 132
strengthening and developing, 64, 87, 88, 97, 100, 104, 181-83
Feng chi acupoint, 60
Fibrinolysis (anti-clotting effect) in blood, 137
"Fiery heart," tranquilizing the, 55
Fingers, flexibility of, 101
Fitness Exercises. *See* Chinese fitness exercises; Flexibility; Strengthening and developing
"Five troubles," the, 54
Flaccid abdominal wall, 165
Flatulence, relief from, 164, 168. *See also* Digestion, improving
Flexibility, 11, 12. *See also* Relaxation; Strengthening and developing; individual parts of the body
ankles, 95
in athletes, 111
in children, 83
fingers, 101
hips, 45, 46, 47, 49, 56, 86, 93, 95, 101, 113
increasing, 9, 11, 20
knees, 45, 95, 101
neck, 99
shoulders, 39, 42
spine, 11, 39, 42, 46, 47, 49, 55, 56, 62, 86, 91, 92, 93, 99, 100, 113, 116
FORWARD THRUST, 114

G

Games and sports, therapeutic
for anxiety and depression, 167, 169-70
for coronary heart disease, 139
following brain concussion, 173
for hypertension, 121, 124, 128
injuries, preventing, 111, 117
for paraplegia, 180-81, 186
Gastrointestinal problems, 159-65. *See also* Digestion, improving;

INDEX

Indigestion; Peptic ulcer; Stomach
bowel illness, 159, 163
Chi Kung for, 159, 160, 163
Chi Kung for the Internal Organs for, 74
constipation, 159-64, 165
diet and, 159, 164
emotional state and, 163
gastroptosis, 164-65
indigestion, 159
massage for, 159, 160, 163
peptic ulcer, 159
psychological state and, 163
obesity, 11, 159
stomach illness, 159
Gluteal muscles, exercises for, 184-85
Gums. *See* Periodontitis

H

HALF-SITTING AND RELAXING, 108
HALF-SQUATTING, 101
Hamstrings, developing, 62
HANDLING TWO CHESTNUTS WITH ONE HAND, 101
Hands
numbness, 132
Strengthening and developing, 45, 177
HANGING AND SWINGING, 116
Head
exercise for hypertension, 126
massage, 60, 129, 154
Headache
relief from, 20, 60, 121, 129, 164, 169, 173
as side effect of *Chi Kung*, 69
as side effect of *Yi Jin Jing*, 35
Heart. *See also* Angina pectoris; Cardiorespiratory fitness; Coronary heart disease; Palpitation
attack
exercises for, 155-57

prevention, 135
Tai Chi Chuan and, 135
treatment, 136-37, 140
disease, 135-57
Chi Kung for Fitness and, 70
lack of activity and, 89
strengthening, 8, 11, 54, 84, 121, 122

Heartburn, relief from, 164
HEAVING, 37
Hemiplegia, exercises for, 175, 176-77
Hiking and hill climbing, 127, 128, 138
Hips
flexibility, 45, 46, 47, 49, 56, 86, 93, 95, 101, 113
strengthening and developing, 114, 183-86
HITTING THE BEAN BAG, 84
HUNGRY TIGER JUMPING TOWARDS THE FOOD, THE, 45
Hypertension, 8, 35, 45, 46, 47, 54, 121-29. *See also* Circulation
arteriosclerosis and, 131, 132, 134
balance and, 124
coordination and, 124
coronary heart disease and, 139
exercises for, 121-29
benefits, 121-24
Breathing exercise, 78, 125
Chi Kung, 121, 122-24
Chi Kung for Fitness, 70
Chi Kung for Relaxation, 122
Head exercise, 126
Relaxation exercise, 125
Sideward stretch, 126
Tai Chi Chuan, 19, 20, 121, 124
Upward stretch, 127
Walking, 127
games and, 121, 128
massage for, 104, 121, 124, 129
and the nervous system, 123-24
principle of descent, 123

199

INDEX

treatment, 19, 20, 104, 121-29
Yi Jin Jing and, 35
Hyperventilation, 68

I

Ilio-psoas, exercises for, 183-84
Imagination, in exercises. *See* Mental concentration; Visualization
INCREASING THE VITAL ENERGY BY TIGHTENING THE FISTS AND GAZING STERNLY, 57
Indigestion. *See also* Digestion, improving
  flaccid abdominal wall and, 165
  relief from, 63, 164
  treatment, 159
Insomnia, 171-72. *See also* Relaxation
  arteriosclerosis and, 132
  breathing for, 172
  Chi Kung for Sleep, 172
  emotional state and, 171
  exercises for, 55, 171-72
  massage for, 104, 172
  Tai Chi Chuan for, 171
  treatment, 20, 64, 121, 132, 171
Internal organs, massage of, 65
Intervertebral disk problems. *See* Disk problems
Ischemia (deficient blood supply), 132, 136, 178

J

Jogging, 11, 20
  for anxiety and depression, 167, 168, 169-70
  for coronary heart disease, 135, 138, 139
  for gastrointestinal problems, 159, 160, 162, 163
  for hypertension, 128
  to control weight, 11

K

KEEPING ALL DISEASES AWAY BY RAISING THE HEELS SEVEN TIMES, 58
KICKING, 95
Kidneys, 54
KNEE BENDING, 160
KNEE BENDING AND RELAXING, 107
Knees
  degeneration of cartilage, 43
  flexibility, 45, 95, 101
  massage, 118, 129
  strengthening and developing, 35, 43, 92, 104, 111, 112, 115, 178, 181-82

L

LEG RAISING, 161
Legs. *See also* Ankles; Calves; Feet; Knees; Thighs
  circulation, 64, 95
  numbness as a side effect of *Chi Kung,* 68
  reducing of swelling in, 105, 110
  relief from pain in, 187
  strengthening and developing, 49, 62, 101, 103, 115, 122, 123
LIFTING THE PLATES, 43
Lipid levels
  and arteriosclerosis, 131
  and coronary heart disease, 137
Liver, 54
Longevity, 9, 65
Lumbar disk problems. *See* Disk problems
Lungs. *See also* Breathing
  developing, 8, 11, 12, 54, 84, 121

M

MAKING A GESTURE OF RESPECT WITH BOTH HANDS FACING THE CHEST, 36
Massage, 8, 17-18, 59, 102-4. *See also* Acupuncture points, massage of
  abdomen, 63, 102, 163

INDEX

for anxiety and depression, 168, 169
arms, 117
for arteriosclerosis, 132, 134
for athletes, 111, 117-18
back, 63
following brain concussion, 173
and Chinese exercise therapy, 8
for constipation, 160, 163
for coronary heart disease, 154
for the elderly, 102-4
eyes, 88
face, 60, 129, 154
feet, 64, 104, 129
for gastrointestinal problems, 159
head, 129, 154
for hypertension, 121, 124, 129
for insomnia, 172
internal organs, 65
knees, 118, 129
neck, 60, 129, 154
for paralysis, 175, 176, 181
for polio, 181
shoulders, 118
for sciatica and lumbar disk problems, 187
stomach, 50
thighs, 117
Medication, reliance on, 7
for hypertension, 122
Meditation. *See* Mental concentration; Visualization
Mental concentration, 8, 17, 19, 167. *See also* Visualization
for anxiety and depression, 167, 168
in *Chi Kung*, 65, 66, 67, 68, 69-70, 72-73, 75
for hypertension, 122, 124
for insomnia, 172
in *Tai Chi Chuan*, 20, 21
Yi Jin Jing for, 35, 36, 37, 38, 39, 40-41, 42, 43
Mental relaxation. *See* Relaxation

Mental stress. *See* Anxiety and depression; Emotional state; Relaxation
Metabolism. *See also* Digestion, improving
diseases, 159
improving, 137
MONKEY PLAY, 85
MOVING THE TONGUE AROUND, 60
Muscles, 8, 11. *See also* Flexibility; Massage; Strengthening and developing; individual parts of the body
atrophy, 181
flaccid, 175
spastic, 175
tone, 11, 35
weakness, 132, 173
Muscle strengthening exercises. *See* Strengthening and developing; *Yi Jin Jing*
Musculoskeletal problems
in the elderly, 97-104
in the sedentary, 89-95

N

Neck
flexibility of, 99
massage, 60, 129, 154
preventing stiffness, 11, 39, 42, 91, 99
relief from pain, 35, 39, 42
strengthening and developing, 45, 54, 97
Nervous system, 123-24. *See also* Emotional state; Relaxation
Neuromuscular tension, reducing, 169
Nocturnal emissions, relief from, 63

O

Obesity, 7, 159. *See also* Diet
Occupational therapy for paralysis, 177

INDEX

Old form *Tai Chi Chuan.* See *Tai Chi Chuan*
Overeating, 159
   relief from, 54

P

Palpitation
   relief from, 64, 121
   as side effect of *Chi Kung,* 68–69
Palsies. *See* Polio
Paralysis. *See also* Hemiplegia; Paraplegia; Polio
   acupuncture for, 175
   benefits of exercises for, 175
   duration of exercises, 175
   functional training exercises, 175
   massage for, 175
   spinal cord injury, 175
   stroke, 175
   walking, 175
Paraplegia
   causes of, 177
   circulation and, 178
   defined, 177
   exercises for, 175, 177–80
      benefits, 177–78
   faintness and, 178
   games for, 180–81
   ischemia and, 178
   scoliosis and, 181
   surgical intervention, 178
   therapeutic sports, 180
   treatment, 177
PELVIC ROCKING, 106
Pelvis
   relaxation of, 107, 108, 109
   relief from pressure on, 105
Peptic ulcer. *See also* Gastrointestinal problems; Relaxation; Stomach
   Chi Kung for the Internal Organs for, 74
   Exercise with *Tai Chi* stick for, 79
   treatment, 8, 159

Periarthritis, 61. *See also* Arthritis
Periodontitis, 60
Peripheral ischemia. *See* Ischemia
Peroneal muscle, developing, 182–83
Phobias, relief from, 167. *See also* Anxiety and depression; Emotional state; Relaxation
Physical Fitness. *See Ba Duan Jin;* Chinese fitness exercises; Flexibility; Strengthening and developing; *Yi Jin Jing;* individual parts of the body
Physical relaxation. *See* Relaxation
PICKING UP BEANS, 92
Polio
   causes of, 181
   exercises for, 181–86
   massage for, 181
   games for, 186
Popliteal fossa, massage of, 129
Posture. *See also* Back; Spine
   in *Chi Kung,* 65
   for children, 83
   faulty, 165
   improving, 9, 11, 35, 36, 37, 38, 49, 50, 58, 87
Pregnant women
   exercises for, 105–10
      benefits, 11, 105
      Abdominal breathing, 106
      Half-sitting and relaxing, 108
      Knee bending and relaxing, 107
      Pelvic rocking, 106
      Squatting and relaxing, 109
      Stretching and relaxing, 110
      Tailor sitting (sitting cross-legged) and rhythmic breathing, 108
      Walking, 109
Preventive health and lifestyle, 7, 8, 9, 136
Psychological state. *See* Anxiety and depression; Emotional state;

INDEX

Mental concentration; Relaxation
Psychosomatic illness, 8. *See also* Anxiety and depression; *Chi Kung;* Emotional state; Hypertension; Mental concentration; Relaxation
Psychoneuroses, 8. *See also* Anxiety and depression; Emotional state; Relaxation
Chi Kung for Fitness for, 70
Exercise with *Tai Chi* stick for, 79
PULLING THE EAR, 42
PULLING THE TAILS OF NINE OXEN, 40-41
Pulmonary emphysema, 70. *See* Emphysema
PUSHING THE MOUNTAIN, 41
PUSHING TOWARDS THE SKY (SHIER DUAN JIN), 61
PUSHING TOWARDS THE SKY (YI JIN JING), 38
PUSHING WITH THE HANDS WHILE RIDING A HORSE, 92

Q

Quadriceps, 112
 developing, 181-82
Quietness training in *Chi Kung*, 66, 72-73, 75. *See also* Relaxation

R

REACHING THE STARS, 39
REGULATING THE INTERNAL ORGANS BY RAISING BOTH HANDS TO THE SKY, 50
REGULATING THE SPLEEN AND STOMACH BY RAISING THE HAND UPWARD, 53
Relaxation, 7-9, 11, 17, 20, 116. *See also* Breathing; Emotional state; Mental concentration
 for anxiety and depression, 167-68
 Ba Duan Jin for, 54, 55
 following brain concussion, 173

Chi Kung for, 64, 65, 66, 69-70, 72-73, 75
 in coronary heart disease, 135, 137
 exercise with the *Tai Chi* stick for, 79
 in hypertension, 121, 122, 123-24, 125
 in insomnia, 171-72
 in pregnancy, 106, 107, 108, 109
 Tai Chi Chuan for, 19, 20
 Yi Jin Jing for, 36
RELAXING THE WAIST AND TAPPING THE BODY, 116-17
Respiration. *See* Breathing
Restlessness, 55. *See also* Relaxation
Rheumatism, treatment of, 20, 54
Rib pain, as side effect of *Chi Kung*, 68
RIDING A HORSE, 112
ROPE JUMPING, 84
Rowing, 162
ROWING, 100
Running. *See* Jogging

S

Saliva, secretion of, 60
Sciatica, 187-91. *See also* Back; Backache; Posture; Spine
 causes, 187
 defined, 187
 disk problems and, 191
 exercises for, 188-91
  benefits, 187
 inflammation of nerves, 187
 lumbosacral arthritis, 187
 massage for, 187
 sacroiliac arthritis, 187
 sciatic neuritis, 187
 symptoms, 191
 treatment, 191
Scoliosis, 87, 181
Sedentary, the, 89-95
 arteriosclerosis and, 131
 coronary heart disease and, 89
 exercises for, 90-95

INDEX

benefits, 11, 89
Kicking, 95
Picking up beans, 92
Pushing with the hands while riding a horse, 92
Spreading the "wings," 94
Swaying from the waist and hips, 93
Swinging the arms, 90
Twisting the trunk and looking backward, 91
Walking like the wind, 94
Self-administered massage. *See* Acupuncture points, massage of; Massage
Self-esteem and confidence, enhancing, 11, 19, 169. *See also* Well-being, promoting
Self-control, increasing, 19
"Seven disorders," the, 54
Shen shu acupoint, 63, 103
Shier Duan Jin (Twelve fine exercises), 59–64
  for the chronically ill, 59
  for the elderly, 59
  exercises, 60–64
    benefits, 11, 12, 59
    Beating the "drum of heaven," 60
    Bending the trunk with the hands touching the feet, 62
    Biting the teeth, 60
    Drawing a bow, 62
    Moving the tongue around, 60
    Pushing towards the sky, 61
    Stretching the legs, 64
    Stroking the *dan tian* (field of pills), 63
    Stroking the *shen shu* (kidney point), 63
    Stroking the *yung chuan*, 64
    "Washing" the face, 60
    Winding the pulley, 61

SHOOTING THE EAGLE BY DRAWING THE BOW WITH THE HANDS, 51–52
Shoulders
  flexibility, 39, 42
  massage, 118
  strengthening and developing, 51, 53, 61, 62, 90, 98, 114, 178, 180, 185
Simplified *Tai Chi Chuan*. *See Tai Chi Chuan*
Sit ups, 162
Skin, circulation in, 60
Sleep, lack of. *See* Insomnia
Spine. *See also* Back; Backache; Posture
  curvature of, 87, 165, 181
  flexibility of, 11, 39, 42, 46, 47, 49, 55, 56, 62, 86, 91, 92, 93, 99, 100, 113, 116
  injury to, 175, 177
  and surgical intervention, 178
"Spiritual exercise," 167
Spleen, 53, 54
Sports. *See* Athletes; Games and sports, therapeutic
SPREADING THE "WINGS," 94
SQUATTING AND RELAXING, 109
Stamina, increasing, 12. *See also* Chinese fitness exercises; Chinese therapeutic exercises; Strengthening and developing
Standing Chi Kung and hypertension, 122–23
Stomach. *See also* Digestion, improving; Indigestion; Peptic ulcer
  illness, prevention of, 159
  massage, 50
  strengthening and developing, 164
Strengthening and developing, 11, 35. *See also Ba Duan Jin;* Chinese fitness exercises; Flexibility; Massage; *Yi Jin Jing;* individual parts of body
  abdomen, 115, 160–62, 164, 165, 185

INDEX

ankles, 88, 118
arms, 39, 41, 44, 45, 49, 53, 57, 84, 92, 101, 114, 178, 185
back, 41, 53, 62, 87, 111, 115, 178, 180, 185
buttocks, 184-85
calves, 58, 87
chest, 36, 49, 51, 61, 62, 94
for coronary heart disease, 135, 136, 139, 163
feet, 64, 87, 88, 97, 100, 104, 181-83
hands, 45, 177
heart, 11, 54, 84, 121, 122
hips, 114, 183-86
knees, 35, 43, 92, 104, 111, 112, 115, 178, 181-82
legs, 49, 62, 101, 103, 115, 122, 123
neck, 45
for polio, 181-86
shoulders, 51, 53, 61, 62, 90, 98, 114, 178, 180, 185
stomach, 164
thighs, 35, 43, 51, 55, 114
STRENGTHENING THE LOINS AND KIDNEYS BY BENDING FORWARD WITH HANDS TOUCHING THE FEET, 56
Stretching exercises, 44, 62, 64, 110, 116, 126-27, 141, 142, 148-49. *See also* Yi Jin Jing; and individual exercises
STRETCHING THE ARMS, 44
STRETCHING THE LEGS, 64
STRETCHING AND RELAXING, 110
Stress, relief from. *See* Anxiety and depression; Mental concentration; Relaxation
Stroke, exercises following, 175
SWALLOW FLYING, 115
SWAYING FROM THE WAIST AND HIPS, 93
Swimming
  and coronary heart disease, 139
  and hypertension, 121, 124, 127
SWINGING THE ARMS, 90, 98

Symbolism in Chinese exercises, 8, 17. *See also* Visualization
Sympathetic nervous system. *See* Nervous system
Syncope. *See* Faintness

T

Tai Chi Chuan, 19-34
  for anxiety and depression, 168
  for arteriosclerosis, 132
  benefits of, 7, 9, 11, 19-21
  breathing and, 20, 21, 165
  circulation and, 20
  for coronary heart disease, 135, 139
  defined, 19
  digestion and, 20
  how to practice, 20-22
  for hypertension, 19, 121, 124
  for insomnia, 171
  intensity of, 20-21
  mental concentration and, 20, 21
  need for a teacher, 22
  Old form, 124
  popularity of, 21
  physical relaxation and, 21
  principles of, 21-22
  Simplified, 21, 124
  illustrated, 23-34
Tai Chi stick, exercise with
  benefits, 79
  exercises, 79-80
    Circling at a resting position, 79
    Circling while moving the legs up and down, 79
    Circling while walking, 80
  possible side effects of, 80
TAILOR SITTING AND RHYTHMIC BREATHING, 108
Tao yin, 20, 59
Teeth. *See* Periodontitis
Tension, relief from, 168. *See also* Anxiety and depression;

INDEX

Emotional state; Flexibility; Mental concentration; Relaxation
Terrain cure, 138
Therapeutic exercise. *See* Chinese therapeutic exercises
Thighs
  massage of, 117
  strengthening and developing, 35, 43, 51, 55, 114
TIGER WALKING, 86, 113
TIP-TOE WALKING, 87
Traditional Chinese exercises, 11, 12, 13, 15-80
  benefits of, 7-13, 17, 167-68
  principles of, 17-18
  Ba Duan Jin (Eight fine exercises), 49-58
  Breathing exercise, 78
  Chi Kung (Invigorating exercises), 65-75, 122, 123, 139, 163, 164-65, 168-69, 172
  Shier Duan Jin (Twelve fine exercises), 59-64
  Tai Chi Chuan, 19-34, 124, 135, 139, 168, 171
  Tai Chi stick, exercise with, 79-80
  Yi Jin Jing, 35-47
TRANQUILIZING THE FIERY HEART BY TURNING THE HEAD AROUND AND SWINGING THE HIPS, 55
TWISTING THE TRUNK AND LOOKING BACKWARD, 91

V

Vertigo, 133, 164, 169, 173
Viral hepatitis, 74
Vision, improving, 88
Visualization, 17. *See also* Mental concentration
  for athletes, 112, 113, 115
  in *Ba Duan Jin*, 51-52, 54, 57
  for children, 85, 86, 87

for the elderly, 99, 100
for the sedentary, 92, 94
in *Shier Duan Jin*, 60, 61, 62
in *Tai Chi Chuan*, 21, 22
in *Yi Jin Jing*. *See* each of the exercises, 35-47
Vitality, enhancing, 103. *See Chi Kung;* Chinese fitness exercises; Well-being, promoting

W

Walking, 11, 94, 102
  for anxiety and depression, 169
  for arteriosclerosis, 132
  for constipation, 162
  for coronary heart disease, 11, 138, 139, 141, 152, 156
  for heart attack, 156
  for hypertension, 121, 124, 127, 128
  for insomnia, 171
  for paralysis, 175, 176, 177, 179-80
  for polio, 179-80, 185, 186
  for pregnant women, 109
  to control weight, 11
WALKING LIKE THE WIND, 94
WALKING AND MASSAGING THE ABDOMEN, 102
WALL PUSHING, 115
"WASHING" THE FACE, 60
Weight control, 11. *See also* Diet; Obesity; Overeating
Well-being, promoting, 54, 59-64, 78, 90, 98, 103. *See also* Mental concentration; Relaxation; Self-esteem and confidence
WINDING THE PULLEY, 61
WORM WRIGGLING, 87

Y

Yi Jin Jing (Muscle strengthening exercises), 9, 11, 13, 35-47

INDEX

as body/mind exercises, 8, 36–47
benefits of, 11
exercises, 36–47
   Bending forward, 47
   Bowing, 46
   Heaving, 37
   The hungry tiger jumping towards the food, 45
   Lifting the plates, 43
   Making a gesture of respect with both hands facing the chest, 36
   Pulling the ear, 42
   Pulling the tails of nine oxen, 40–41
   Pushing the mountain, 41
   Pushing towards the sky, 38
   Reaching the stars, 39
   Stretching the arms, 44
mental concentration in, 35, 36
principles of, 35
as stretching exercise, 36–38
Yin and *Yang*, 19
Yung chuan acupoint, 64, 104, 129, 172